The Veterinarian

by Chas. J. Korinek

FOREWORD

This treatise on the diseases of domestic animals has been written with the primary purpose of placing in the hands of stock owners, a book of practical worth; hence, all technical language or terms, as used by the professional veterinarian, have been eliminated and only such language used as all may read and understand.

The treatment suggested in each case is one I have used and found efficient in my many years of practice.

If my readers will study and follow these directions carefully, they will save themselves much unnecessary loss. My confidence in this accomplishment is my reward for my labor in behalf of our dumb friends--the domestic animals.
THE AUTHOR

CONTENTS

DISEASES OF THE HORSE

Causes, Symptoms and Treatments

LOCATION OF PARTS OF THE HORSE 1. Mouth 2. Nostrils 3. Nose 4. Face 5. Eyes 6. Forehead 7. Ears 8. Poll 9. Throat latch 10. Jaw 11. Chin 12. Windpipe 13. Neck 14. Crest 15. Withers 16. Shoulder bed 17. Chest 18. Shoulders 19. Forearm 20. Knees 21. Cannon 22. Fetlocks 23. Pasterns 24. Feet 25. Feather 25-1/2. Elbow 26. Flank 27. Heart Girth 28. Back 29. Loin 30. Hip bone 31. Coupling 32. Ribs 33. Belly 34. Rear Flank 35. Stifle 36. Thigh 37. Buttocks 38. Croup 39. Tail 40. Quarters 41. Gaskin or Lower Thigh 42. Hocks

CHAPTER I

ABORTION IN MARES

CAUSE: Quality and quantity of food, poorly lighted, ventilated or drained stables, mare falling or slipping, sprains, kicks, hard, fast work or eating poisonous vegetation.

SYMPTOMS: Mare will show signs of colic, the outer portion of the womb will be swollen, and if the colicky symptoms continue there will be a watery discharge and the membranes covering the foetus or foal will become noticeable. The animal strains when lying down or getting up.

TREATMENT: Place the animal in comfortable quarters and blanket if chilly. When colicky pains are present treat the same as for spasmodic colic. To stop the straining and labor pains, give Tincture Opii one ounce, placing in gelatin capsule and give with capsule gun every two hours. One to two doses, however, are generally sufficient as the mare will either abort or the dangerous period will have passed. Keep the animal quiet and feed good nutritious food and pure water with chill taken off in small quantities but often. Disinfect the mare's quarters thoroughly. A good general tonic should be used in this condition, one that will strengthen and assist nature to throw off impurities from the blood, such as Sodium Hyposulphite, eight ounces; Potassi Iodide, one ounce. Make into eight powders and give one powder two or three times a day in drinking water.

ABSCESS

CAUSE: Bruises and injuries. Abscesses are also seen in complications with various diseases, perhaps the most common being distemper, laryngitis, etc.

SYMPTOMS: Symptoms will vary, of course, according to the development of the disease. It may not be noticed at first, but upon careful examination small tortuous lines will be observed running from the point of irritation. In many cases a swelling is noticed which is hot, painful and throbbing and enlarges rapidly. In two or three days the soreness and heat gradually subside, but the abscess continues to grow. The hair falls from the affected parts and in a short time the abscess discharges, and the cavity gradually fills up and heals by granulation.

TREATMENT: In all cases hasten the repairing process as much as possible by applying hot water packs or hot bran, flaxseed or vegetable poultices. It is common with veterinarians to lance an abscess as soon as possible, but this requires skill and practice. I could not advise stockowners to perform this operation, as it requires exact knowledge of anatomy. It will usually be found a safe plan to encourage the full ripening of an abscess and allow it to open of its own accord, as it will heal much better and quicker and you take no chances of infection with an instrument. When opened do not squeeze the abscess to any extent, but press gently with clean hands or cloth, to remove the clot, and after this simply keep open by washing the abscess with a three per cent Carbolic Acid solution or Bichloride of Mercury, one part to one thousand parts of water. When an animal has abscesses it is well to give the following blood purifiers or internal antiseptics: Hyposulphite of Soda, eight ounces; Potassi Iodide, one ounce. Mix well and make into eight powders and give one powder twice daily in drinking water, or place in gelatin capsule and administer with capsule gun. This prescription will prevent the absorption of impurities from the abscess into the blood.

ANEMIA

CAUSE: Insufficient quality and quantity of food, insanitary surroundings, overwork, lack of exercise, drains on the system from acute or chronic diseases, worms; and can also be brought about by excessive heat, cold or pressure and lessening of the calibre of the arteries, poisons in the blood, suppurating wounds, repeated purging or bleedings.

SYMPTOMS: The visible mucous membranes of the nose, eyes and mouth are pale and sometimes have a yellow appearance. There is weakness, temperature of the body is lower than normal; pulse weak, legs cold to the feet, cold sweats are often present, breathing is quickened, especially in its last stages, animals tire easily, appetite and digestion become poor, swelling of the legs and the under surface of the abdomen, sheath and udder; the skin becomes rough and dry.

TREATMENT: Remove the cause if possible in its first stages, or when first noticed. Give a physic of Calomel, two scruples; Aloin, two drams; Pulv. Gentian, two drams; Ginger, two drams. Place in gelatin capsule and give at one dose with capsule gun. Also, administer the following: Arsenious Acid, one dram; Ferri Sulphate, three ounces; Pulv. Gentian, three ounces; Pulv. Fenugreek Seed, three ounces, and Pulv. Anise Seed, three ounces. Mix well and make into twenty powders. Give one powder three times a day in feed, or place in gelatin capsule and give with capsule gun. Endeavor to build up the condition of the animal by the proper quantity and quality of food. Give pure water to drink, also provide sanitary conditions, as pure air, sunlight if possible. Turn out to grass when the weather is favorable. This treatment should be continued until the animal shows sign of improvement. However, the administration of physics should be given with great care so as not to produce superpurgation of the bowels (scours), as physics in this condition would tend to weaken the animal.

It is to be borne in mind that pure water and nourishing food play a very important part in the treatment of Anemia.

APHTHAE

(Sore mouth and tongue--Pustular Stomatitis)

CAUSE: Superficial eruptions of the mucous membranes of the mouth and tongue. Frequently seen during convalescence of intermittent fever. This condition may also follow diseases of the digestive system, as Indigestion, etc., due to the blood absorbing toxic materials which break out in the form of pustules about the mouth and the whole alimentary canal (stomach and intestines).

SYMPTOMS: The appetite is impaired, the mouth hot, the pulse not much affected as a rule, the temperature is slightly elevated, the animal is unable to masticate, and small vesicles appear and eventually terminate into pustules and burst and discharge a small amount of pus at the parts where the sores are the deepest.

TREATMENT: Remove the cause if possible. Feed clean, soft food that is easily digested, as hot wheat bran mashes and steamed rolled oats, vegetables, etc. For a mouth-wash dissolve the following: One dram of Copper Sulphate, one dram of Chlorate of Potash, one dram of Boracic Acid in clean hot water, and syringe out the mouth two or three times a day. To the drinking water add one ounce of Hyposulphite of Soda twice a day. Where the appetite is impaired, administer the following: Pulv. Nux Vomica, Pulv. Gentian Root, Pulv. Iron, Pulv. Nitrate of Potash each two ounces. Mix and make into sixteen capsules and give one capsule three times a day with capsule gun.

AZOTURIA

CAUSE: This disease is usually due to work after a period of idleness, during which the animal has been liberally fed. It is found principally among highly-fed draft horses, and never in animals which are regularly worked. Light breeds of horses are also susceptible to this disease.

SYMPTOMS: Attack is sudden and usually appears when the horse has traveled a short distance after having been stabled for a few days. The characteristic symptoms of this disease in an animal are: Excitability without apparent cause; actions seem to indicate injury of the hind quarters or loins. Animal has a peculiar goose-rumped look, owing to the muscles over the quarters being violently contracted, and are hard on pressure. One hind limb is generally advanced in front of the other, and on attempting to put weight on it, the hind quarters will drop until at times the hocks almost touch the ground. Sometimes a front leg is affected. The breathing is hurried. Animal is bathed in sweat, and is in such agony that it will seize almost anything with its teeth. Although the pulse is hard and frequent, the internal temperature, even in severe cases, seldom rises to any marked extent. The urine is dark-red to dirty-brown color. Owing to the stoppage of the worm-like movement of the bowels, there is generally constipation and retention of the urine. Sometimes the symptoms are milder than here described. In other cases the animal soon falls to the ground and continues to struggle in a delirious, half-paralyzed state until he dies. Sometimes this disease is mistaken for colic or acute indigestion, but it can be readily distinguished by the color of the urine.

TREATMENT: At the first symptom, stop and blanket the animal and let stand from one to three hours. Then move to the nearest shelter, keeping the animal as quiet and comfortable, as possible, as excitement aggravates the disease. Give Aloin, two drams; Ginger, two drams; in capsule, and administer with capsule gun. Also, give the following prescription: Potassi Nitrate, eight ounces; Sodii Bicarbonate, eight ounces; Potassi Iodide, one and one-half ounces. Mix well and make into thirty-two powders. Give one powder in drinking water every four hours, or in capsule, and give with capsule gun. Injections of soap and warm water per rectum are beneficial. Immerse a blanket in hot water and place over loins, then covering with a dry blanket, or, if this is impossible, apply the following liniment: Aqua Ammonia Fort., two ounces; Turpentine, two ounces; Sweet Oil, four ounces, and rub in like a shampoo over the loins. It may be necessary to draw off the urine, which is sometimes retained, and it is best to secure the services of a skilled veterinarian if, such is the case. Allow the animal to drink often, though in small quantities, of pure water with the chill taken off. If he is unable to stand on his feet it is well to turn him from side to side every six hours. It is also advisable to fill bags with hay and place against his shoulders to prevent him from lying flat on his side, as this may cause congestion of the lungs. Avoid drenching--it is dangerous. Should the animal show signs of uneasiness, give one ounce of Potassi Bromide in the drinking water every four hours until the excitement has subsided.

BARRENNESS

(Failure to Breed)

CAUSE: Contraction of the neck of the womb, growths on or in the ovaries, Whites or Leucorrhea. The first is the only form of barrenness which responds readily to treatment.

SYMPTOMS: A mare may come in heat normally, or stay in heat continually, or not come in heat at all.

TREATMENT: Wash the hands in some antiseptic solution, such as Carbolic Acid or Bichloride of Mercury and see that the finger-nails are smooth. Grease the hand and arm with vaseline and proceed to dilate the neck of the womb. It may be difficult at first to insert the finger, but the opening will gradually enlarge. Work slowly and carefully until three fingers may be inserted. Breeding should follow about three hours after the womb has been dilated.

BLEEDING AFTER CASTRATION

If bleeding is from the little artery in the back portion of cord, it will generally stop of its own accord, but if it should continue to bleed for thirty minutes, I throw clean, cold water against the part.

When bleeding is from the large artery in front of the cord, it is considered dangerous. The artery should be tied with a silk thread if possible, or twisted with a pair of forceps. Occasionally the artery cannot be found, in which case the hole in the scrotum should be plugged with a clean cloth saturated with Tincture of Iron, which will clot the blood and thus close the artery.

BLOOD POISONING

(Septicaemia or Pyemia)

CAUSE: By the popular term, "Blood Poison," is meant a state of constitutional disturbance brought on by the entrance of putrid products-- usually from a wound--into the blood. As a rule some pressure or inoculation is necessary for the introduction of poison into the circulation; hence, the necessity of free drainage and thorough disinfection of the wound, and the only hopeful cases are those in which by this means the supply of poison may be cut short.

SYMPTOMS: It is introduced through any wound or abrasion, whether due to injury, disease or by an operation. Signs of septic poison are heat, pain and swelling.

TREATMENT: It is necessary to see that the wound has good drainage, and wash with Carbolic Acid, one tablespoonful to one pint of distilled water or Bichloride of Mercury perhaps is the best in an infected wound. Apply one part to one thousand parts water. Also, give internally, Potassi Iodide, one ounce; Sodii Hyposulphite, eight ounces. Make into eight powders and give one powder two or three times a day in their drinking water or in capsule, and give with capsule gun. This is an intestinal antiseptic which is very valuable in the treatment of Blood Poisoning. Feed soft, laxative food and green grass, if possible.

BONE SPAVIN

CAUSE: Sprains of the hock from falling, slipping, jumping, pulling, traveling on uneven roads, falling through bridges, etc.

Since Spavin is due to causes which come into existence after birth, it cannot be regarded as an hereditary disease. Hereditary predisposition, however, is largely accountable for its appearance. In the first place, the process of evolution in the horse, which is a single-toed animal, descended from a five-toed ancestor, predisposes him to suffer from union of the bones of the hock, just as it predisposes him to splints. The weaker the bones of the hock in comparison to the weight of the body the more inclined will the animal naturally be to contract Spavin.

SYMPTOMS: Spasmodic catching up of the spavined limb, the moment the heel of the foot touches the ground, something after the manner of string-halt. At times the stiffness can be observed only when the animal is pushed from one side of the stall to the other. Spavin may often be detected when riding a horse down a steep hill from the fact that he drags the toe.

The time of all others when a spavined horse will be apt to show his lameness will be the day following a hard day's work, and when he makes his first move from the stable in the morning is the proper moment for examination. Therefore, you should be prepared to form judgment quickly in these cases, for the longer the animal is trotted up and down the less lame will he generally become.

We may have a visible sign of Spavin, swelling and hardness of the part, without lameness. If there be heat and tenderness on pressure, lameness will almost always be present. A careful comparison should be made of the hocks.

TREATMENT: An important factor in treating Spavin is keeping the animal quiet. This can be accomplished by placing the animal in a very narrow stall, carrying his feed and drinking water for a month or six weeks, and apply the following ointment: Red Iodide of Mercury, two drams; Pulverized Cantharides, three drams; Turpentine, thirty minims; Pine Tar, two drams; lard, two ounces. Mix well and rub in well for twenty minutes every forty-eight hours until three applications have been applied. Repeat this treatment again in two weeks, and grease well with lard.

To cure a bone spavin it is necessary to unite two or more bones of the hock, and a fractured bone cannot unite if moved frequently. The same thing exists in bone spavin as in a fractured bone, only we have no ragged edges like that of a fractured bone to unite; therefore, keep the animal quiet. The younger the animal the easier the spavin is to treat, because the bones hardened with age contain more mineral matter and less flexible animal matter. While treating the animal, feed food that is easily digested.

BOG SPAVIN

CAUSE: Faulty conformation, slipping, falling through a bridge or culvert; large loosely built draft horses are prone to this blemish. Bog Spavin is hereditary, and you should, therefore, select a good type of animal for breeding purposes.

SYMPTOMS: A puffy swelling located in front and on the inside of the hock, varying from the size of a walnut to that of a man's fist. It very seldom causes lameness, but is a serious disfigurement and blemish.

TREATMENT: Treatment is not satisfactory unless taken in its first stages and when the animal is young. If there is heat, pain and swelling, apply cold water or ice packs until the inflammation has left the parts. Then use the following prescription: Tincture of Iodine, two ounces; Gum Camphor, two ounces; Gasolene, one pint. Mix and shake well before applying with a nail or tooth brush twice a week.

I may add that I have derived some wonderful results in treatment of Bog Spavin with the above mentioned prescription in both young and old animals, and perhaps it will be well to use it on both young and old animals in both acute and chronic forms of Bog Spavin.

BOTS

(Gastrophilis)

Effect of Bots on the Health of Horses

Although the presence of bots inside of a horse can be of no possible advantage to him, their presence, when in small numbers, as a rule produce very little or no ill effect in the horse, but if their number be large they cannot help being a source of debility and irritation. In practically all cases they produce indigestion, especially among young horses, also loss of condition, colic and even death.

CAUSE: By the bot flies, which lay their eggs during the autumn on the skin and hair of the horses. These eggs on becoming hatched (in from 20 to 25 days) produce small worms which irritate the skin by their movements and thus cause the horse to lick them off and to take them into his mouth, with the result that they gain access to various parts of the intestinal canal. The bot having selected its place of residence, attaches itself to the membranes lining the stomach and intestines, and derives its sustenance during its stay from the wound made by its hooks. In the summer the larva, after living inside the horse for about ten months, quits its hold and is expelled with the feces. Having concealed itself near the surface of the ground it becomes changed into a chrysalis from which the gadfly issues after an inactive existence of from thirty to forty days. The female fly becomes impregnated, lays her eggs on those parts of the horse from which they can be most easily licked off, and thus completes her cycle of existence.

SYMPTOMS: Membranes about the eyes and mouth are very pale, as though the animal had lost a large quantity of blood; they will also be subject to colicky attacks, hair faded, dull, rough appearance, appetite poor and manifests a pot belly.

PREVENTION: The best means of prevention are spraying your horses with the following fly repellant: Crude Carbolic Acid, 10%; Oil of Tar, 25%; Crude Oil, 65%. Mix thoroughly. This prevents the gadfly from depositing her eggs on the animals.

TREATMENT: Withhold all food for twenty-four hours, then administer Oil of Turpentine, one ounce; place in a gelatin capsule and give with capsule gun. Follow this in six hours with a physic consisting of Aloin, two drams; Ginger, two drams. Place in a gelatin capsule and give with capsule gun. Repeat the above treatment in a week or ten days to insure the expulsion of Bots that might have escaped the first treatment.

BRONCHITIS

CAUSE: It may be the result of debility, constitutional diseases, inhalation of impure air, smoke, or gases. Sometimes brought on by drenching by the escape of liquid into the windpipe; remember, a horse cannot breathe through his mouth. It may also be caused by sudden chill, foreign bodies in windpipe, micro organisms, or it may be associated with influenza, glanders, lung fever, etc.

SYMPTOMS: Sore throat, loss of appetite, thirst, animal appears dull, membranes of the mouth, eyes and nose are reddened; urine is scanty and highly colored; cough dry and husky. After two or three days the cough becomes looser and, a frothy, sticky mucus of a yellowish color is present. This gradually becomes pus-like, after which the animal seems somewhat relieved. In the first stages the pulse is soft and weak, but frequently the temperature is high, ranging from 105 to 106 degrees F.; the breathing is quick and more or less difficult.

TREATMENT: Place the horse in a clean, comfortable, well ventilated stall, exclude drafts, blanket if the weather is chilly. Also, hand rub the legs and bandage them. Inhalations from steam of hot water and Turpentine are beneficial. Also administer Chlorate of Potassi, two ounces; Nitrate of Potash, two ounces; Tannic Acid, one ounce. Mix this with a pint of black-strap molasses and give about one tablespoonful well back on the tongue with a wooden paddle every six hours. In severe attacks of Bronchitis it is well to apply a liniment consisting of Turpentine, Aqua-Ammonia Fort., and raw Linseed Oil, each four ounces; mix well and apply to the throat and down the windpipe once or twice a day. The animal should be fed on soft food, such as hot bran mashes, grass, carrots, kale, apples or steamed rolled oats. After the acute symptoms of the disease disappear, give Pulverized Gentian Root, one ounce; Nux Vomica, two ounces; Nitrate of Potash, three ounces; Pulverized Fenugreek Seed, six ounces. Mix and give one tablespoonful three times a day in the feed or in a gelatin capsule and administer with a capsule gun.

CAPPED KNEE

CAUSE: Bruises from pawing or striking objects with the knee, falling on the ground, etc., are perhaps the most common causes.

SYMPTOMS: It may be a simple bruise, or it may be a severe wound. There is always swelling, heat and pain present. The joint becomes stiff and interferes with the movement of the leg. Under careful treatment the swelling and enlargement disappear.

TREATMENT: Relieve the inflammation and clean the wound by fomenting with hot water, to which add a few drops of Carbolic Acid. If the wound is very large, trim off the ragged edges with a pair of scissors and apply the following: Boracic Acid, two ounces; Iodoform, one ounce; Tannic Acid, one ounce. Powder finely, mix and apply two or three times a day. If the skin is not broken, apply cold water or ice packs until the inflammation has subsided; then use the following: Tincture of Iodine, one ounce; Camphor, two ounces, and Gasolene, eight ounces. Apply with nail or toothbrush every thirty-six hours until the enlargement has disappeared.

CAPPED HOCK

CAUSE: Some horses have the habit of rubbing or striking their hocks against the partition of their stalls. May also be produced by kicks from other horses, or hocks may be bruised by the singletree.

SYMPTOMS: An enlargement at the point of the hock, which may run up along the tendons and muscles of the leg. Repeated injuries cause the hock to enlarge and become flabby, and in some cases it contains a bloody serum or pus.

TREATMENT: Do not attempt to lance the puffy swelling on the point of the hock, as you may produce an open joint, which is very difficult to treat, and chances are that you would lose the animal.

The treatment that I would recommend is to find out the true cause and remove it. When the puffy swelling is swollen, hot and painful, apply cold water or ice packs. When the heat and pain have subsided apply the following: Tincture of Iodine, two ounces; Gum Camphor, two ounces, dissolved in one pint of Gasolene. Shake the contents of the bottle before using each time and apply with a nail or toothbrush every forty-eight hours. This is very penetrating and will remove the enlargement or absorb fluids that might have accumulated from the result of the bruise.

CHOKING

This term applies to obstruction of the gullet as well as that of the windpipe.

CAUSE: Too rapid eating, by which pieces of carrots or other roots, or a quantity of dry food become lodged in the gullet. Although obstructions of the windpipe caused while drenching, or food entering the lungs, will kill an animal in a very short time, obstructions in the gullet may not prove fatal for several days.

TREATMENT: No time should be lost in attempting to remove the obstruction from the gullet. It may be dislodged by gently manipulating the gullet. If unsuccessful in dislodging the obstruction in this manner, secure the services of a competent veterinarian. He will use a probang, an instrument made for this purpose, or inject Sweet or Olive Oil into the gullet with a hypodermic syringe, or give hypodermic injections of Arecoline. In administering drenches with the object of dislodging obstructions in the gullet, you must remember that the liquids used are apt to go the wrong way, that is to say, enter the lungs, and give rise to lung complications, as lung fever, bronchitis, etc. Obstructions of solid substance in the windpipe generally cause death very shortly. When liquids enter the lungs, death is not so apt to occur, as the animal may live several days, and sometimes even get well. They should be treated the same as for lung fever.

CRACKED HEELS

CAUSE: There is little doubt in my mind that ammonia, which is so plentifully found in ill-kept stables, is the chief cause of cracked heels. The action of ammonia on the skin renders it soft and pulpy, and diminishes its strength by separating the layers of which it is composed.

SYMPTOMS: When inflammation is set up in the part, the secretion of natural oil is interfered with and cracks usually occur in the place where the skin becomes wrinkled when the pastern joint is bent. The discharge from cracked heels has an offensive smell. In early stages there is extreme heat and swelling, there is pain and lameness, which usually disappear as the case becomes chronic.

TREATMENT: Keep the affected parts clean as possible, if there is extreme inflammation present. Apply hot poultice made from bran or flaxseed meal. When the inflammation subsides, apply Zinc Ointment twice daily. Before applying each application of ointment, wash with Warm Water and Castile Soap. Feed carrots, green grass, if possible, also hot bran mashes or steam rolled oats each morning. Sometimes it is well to give a physic, and I would recommend Aloin, one and one-half drams; Ginger, two drams. A physic has very good effect in reducing the swelling of the legs.

COFFIN-JOINT LAMENESS

(Navicular Disease)

CAUSE: Driving young animals on hard roads. Always found in the front feet, owing no doubt to the fact the front feet support largely the weight of the body.

SYMPTOMS: The symptoms are very hard to detect. As a rule the animal will point the affected foot when at rest even before there is any lameness present. While at work he apparently goes sound, but when placed in the stable, or when stopped on hard ground, one foot will be set out in front of the other and resting on the toe. It will be noticed that the animal takes a few lame steps and then goes well again. Again he may be lame for a day, or he may leave the stable in the morning apparently well and sound and go lame during the day. In the course of time he will develop a severe case of lameness, which may last for five or six days. These spells are intermittent and finally he becomes permanently lame, and the more he is driven the greater the lameness, and he steps short, wears the toe of the shoe, stumbles, falls on his knees when the road is rough. Sometimes both front feet are affected and the shoulders will be stiff. When put to work he sweats from pain; there will be extreme heat about the foot, and he will flinch from pressure.

Comparatively few recoveries are made from this disease.

TREATMENT: First remove the shoe. If the foot is inflamed, poultice with hot bran or flaxseed meal. After the inflammation disappears, clean the foot well, clip the hair from around the top of the hoof and use the following: Red Iodide of Mercury, two drams; Pulverized Cantharides, four drams; Turpentine, thirty drops; Lard, two ounces. Mix well and apply every forty-eight hours, rubbing in well for twenty minutes each time. After three or four applications have been applied, turn the animal out to pasture. Repeat this treatment again in a month or so. Animals affected with this disease should be put to slow and easy work on soft ground, and carefully shod. This disease is unsatisfactorily treated and only a few cases recover when the best care is taken.

CORNS

CAUSE: Dry feet, increased pressure from ill fitting shoes, or high heeled shoes, which tend to contract the heels and produce corns. Wide flat feet are predisposed to bruises which terminate in corns.

SYMPTOMS: Lameness, or as the old saying goes, "The animal will go tenderfooted." When standing the animal is generally very restless, they paw their bedding behind them at night. Tapping or pressure on the foot will assist in locating a corn.

TREATMENT: Discover the true cause of the corn and remove it if possible. Take away all pressure from over the corn and turn the animal out in some damp pasture. If this cannot be done, put on a flat "bar" shoe, packing the sole of the foot with Pine Tar and Oakum; then place a leather between the foot and shoe. Repeat this application every two weeks, as this will keep the sole soft and flexible, and with proper shoeing your animal will be relieved of corns.

Frequently coffin-joint lameness or navicular disease is mistaken for corns.

CONSTIPATION

CAUSE: Indigestible foods, irregular feeding, lack of, or too much, exercise, insufficient secretion of digestive materials, strictures, ruptures, paralysis, worms, folding and twisting of the intestines, which frequently occurs in old age.

SYMPTOMS: The animal cannot expel the contents of the intestines, which frequently causes colicky pains. Death from this form of constipation is generally due to rupture of the intestines, when due to indigestible foods or irregular feeding. Lack of, or too much, exercise seldom produces death, although the animal may not pass any fecal matter for a week.

TREATMENT: Give a capsule containing Aloin, two drams, and Pulverized Ginger, two drams, every eighteen hours until the animal has a movement of the bowels. Then give the following tonic: Pulverized Nux Vomica, two ounces; Pulverized Gentian Root, two ounces; Pulverized Fenugreek Seed, four ounces. Mix well and give one tablespoonful in feed three times a day. If the animal refuses to eat it in the feed, place one tablespoonful in gelatin capsule and administer with capsule gun. This will stimulate the worm-like movement of the bowels and strengthen the heart action.

Give the animal all the water it will drink. If the water is cold, take the chill off by warming or adding warm water. If the animal will eat, feed food that is easily digested, such as grass, carrots, turnips, potatoes and apples, but do not feed too large a quantity at one time. Hot bran mashes or steamed rolled oats are very nourishing and easily digested. Rectal injections of Soap and Turpentine in small quantities, added to warm water, are very beneficial, and I would recommend their use. It is advisable to elevate the animal's hind parts when giving rectal injections, as compelling the animal to stand with its head lower than its hind parts will cause the animal to retain the injection much longer, consequently it does its intended work much better.

If due to worms, fast the animal for twenty-four hours and give Barbadoes Aloes, three drams; Calomel, one dram; Ferri Sulphate, two drams; Antimony Tartrate, two drams. Place in gelatin capsule and give with capsule gun, This dose should be repeated in ten days to insure the expulsion of newly hatched worms.

COLD

(Nasal Catarrh)

CAUSE: Atmospheric changes common in the spring and fall; animal allowed to chill when standing in a draft, or driven when the system is in a poor condition. It is also produced by inhaling irritating gases, smoke, drenching through the nose, dusty hay or grain that contains infectious matter.

SYMPTOMS: Animal is stupid, does not take food very freely, hair stands and looks dusty, throat becomes sore, pulse is not greatly affected. There may be a slight rise of temperature, say 101 to 103 degrees F. After a day or two there will be a discharge of mucus from the nostrils which may be offensive to the smell. There is generally an increased flow of urine. The breathing is not much affected.

TREATMENT: Make the animal as comfortable as possible by placing in a clean stall with pure air, but avoid drafts. Blanket if the weather is chilly and give the following prescription: Chloride of Potash, two ounces; Nitrate of Potash, four ounces. Mix these well in a pint of Pine Tar and place about one tablespoonful of the mixture as far back on the tongue as possible every six hours. Relief is very certain if this treatment is given in the first stages. If not it will become chronic and terminate into nasal gleet, or lung complications.

COUGH

(Acute and Chronic)

As a cough is a symptom of various diseases, these in addition to the cough should be treated.

KINDS OF COUGH: Many writers give several different varieties, but for sake of convenience I will divide them into two forms, namely: Acute and Chronic.

CAUSE: Acute Coughs are generally due to sudden exposure to cold, drafts and are the forerunning symptom of a disease of the organs of breathing.

Chronic Coughs are associated with, and often a result of, sore throat, lung fever, pleurisy, bronchitis, broken wind, influenza, nasal gleet, catarrh, glanders, heaves and distemper.

TREATMENT: Under each disease of which a cough is a symptom, I have also prescribed to include its suppression. The following prescription is reasonable in price, yet very effective in all forms of cough: Tannic Acid, one ounce; Potassi Chlorate, four ounces; Potassi Nitrate, four ounces. Powder well and mix with Black Strap Molasses, one pint; placing container retaining the above in hot water assists in dissolving. When this is thoroughly mixed add Pine Tar one pint, and place one tablespoonful well back on the tongue with a wooden paddle every three or four hours, according to the severity of the cough.

Sometimes a liniment applied to the throat and windpipe has a good effect, and I would recommend the following on account of its penetrating qualities: Aqua Ammonia Fort., two ounces; Turpentine, two ounces; Raw Linseed Oil, four ounces. Mix and apply twice daily, shaking the contents of the bottle well before using.

COLT CONSTIPATION

CAUSE: Improper digestion of its mother's milk, especially when overheated or not allowed to nurse enough.

SYMPTOMS: The colt appears stupid; does not care to move about, but lies flat on either side and shows signs of great pain.

TREATMENT: Give two tablespoonfuls of Cascara Sagrada. Great care must be exercised in administering the medicine to place it well back on the tongue; do not hold the nose high or some of the liquid may enter the lungs; it is much better to waste some of the medicine. One of the most important factors in the treatment of Colt Constipation is rectal injections; they relieve temperature, gases, and pain, promoting the worm-like action of the bowels and liquefying their contents.

COLT DIARRHOEA

CAUSE: Specific infection, the action of which is favored by insanitary conditions, irregular feeding, or permitting the colt to nurse when the mother is overheated or out of condition.

SYMPTOMS: Frequent watery discharges, sometimes tinged with blood, and as the disease progresses the colt shows signs of great pain. If not treated promptly, the disease will terminate fatally in the course of six or ten days.

TREATMENT: Determine the exact cause, if possible, and remove it. If the colt has not been weaned, attention should at once be given the mare, and if anything is wrong with her, it may be best to take the little patient away from its mother and feed it on cow's milk sweetened with sugar. Give two tablespoonfuls of Castor Oil on the tongue; this will remove the irritant within the bowels. The following prescription is a very reliable remedy: Protan, three ounces; Pulv. Ginger, four drams; Zinc Sulphocarbolates, four grains. Mix and make into twelve powders; give one powder on the tongue every four hours, effecting a cure within a few days. Do not pull the tongue, or hold the head too high. Permit the animal to swallow slowly. Remember that sanitary surroundings are essential in the treatment of all diseases.

CURB

CAUSE: Faulty conformation of the hind legs; that is to say, if an animal has crooked legs, a slight sprain from slipping or jumping will produce Curb. In cases where an animal has well proportioned limbs, and is afflicted with Curb, it is caused by a rupture of the small ligament or cord situated just back of the hock.

SYMPTOMS: A swelling will be noticed on the back part of the hock. At first the animal is lame and the enlargement is hot and painful. After a few days' rest the inflammation will partially subside and the enlargement can be plainly seen. When the animal is walked about he may be very lame at the start, but this will disappear as he is moved.

TREATMENT: When the Curb is hot and painful, it is well to apply ice packs or cold water to the part. When the inflammation subsides, apply Red Iodide of Mercury, two drams; Lard, two ounces. Mix and rub in well for twenty minutes; repeat every forty-eight hours until three applications are applied. If the Curb is of long standing it is more difficult to treat, in which case the above treatment should be repeated again in two or three months. Do not use the animal in drawing heavy loads, or drive on slippery roads, for six months. Give the blister time to strengthen the ruptured tendons. A high-heeled shoe is often valuable in relieving tendons of their tension.

DIARRHOEA

CAUSE: Sudden change of food, frozen food, soft food, unwholesome food, stagnant water, or drinking large quantities of water at one time, purgative medicines, or it may be associated with blood diseases, lung and intestinal affections, or produced by micro-organisms. Many horses, particularly slack loined, slight, "washy" animals, purge if worked or excited, as may be observed among race horses when taken to a race course. Diarrhoea may also be due to worms, or it may be merely an effort on the part of nature to expel some irritant matter from the bowels or from the blood, in which case it should on no account be prematurely checked.

SYMPTOMS: Frequent loose evacuations of the intestines, with or without pronounced abdominal pain; generally, loss of appetite, animal looks gaunt and the hair rough.

TREATMENT: Keep the animal quiet, comfortably stabled and warmly blanketed. Give pure water to drink, often, but in small quantities. If the animal will eat, feed moderately on clean food, as rolled oats and dry bran. Also, give the following prescription: Protan, three ounces; Zinc Sulphocarbolates, ten grains; Creosote, one dram; Powdered Ginger, two ounces; Powdered Gum Catechu, six drams; Powdered Gum Camphor, one-half dram. Mix and make eight powders. Place one powder in gelatin capsule and give with capsule gun, or the same sized dose dissolved in a pint of water and used as a drench. However, be very careful when drenching an animal. It is dangerous. This prescription will not only check the diarrhoea, but will tone the muscular fibres of the intestines which aid in throwing off these irritant matters from the system. If the horse shows colicky pains, administer the same treatment as that recommended for colic. It is well to give the following treatment in the convalescing stages of diarrhoea: Pulv. Gentian Root, four ounces; Ferri Sulphate, four ounces; Pulv. Nux Vomica, four ounces; Pulv. Fenugreek Seed, eight ounces. Mix and give one heaping tablespoonful three times daily in feed. This facilitates digestion by stimulating the flow of gastric juices.

DISTEMPER

CAUSE: Distemper is placed among the germ diseases, and is produced by the Streptococcus of Schutz. It is contagious and a number of animals in the same stable may become affected at the same time. It is supposed to attack an animal but once, but it may be contracted a second time. May occur at any time of the year.

SYMPTOMS: The animal will first appear dull, and show loss of appetite; and the hair will look dull and rough. There will be a watery discharge from the nose, and in a day or so a lump will appear between the jaws; the animal keeps his head in a peculiar position; saliva runs from its mouth; the pulse will be a little faster than normal. The breathing will become more rapid and the lump between the jaws will get larger. This lump, or tumor, may form in other parts of the body, on the shoulder, in the groin, lungs or intestines. It usually causes death if it cannot be absorbed. This is called irregular distemper. A determined effort should be made to draw the lump, or tumor, to a head as soon as possible.

TREATMENT: Place the horse in a clean, well-ventilated and lighted stall, excluding all drafts, blanket the animal, hand rub the legs and bandage them; give inhalations of steam from Hot Water and Turpentine. A good method for heating water for this purpose is to place hot stones or bricks in the water and Turpentine. This will relieve the hard breathing. Remember a horse cannot breathe through his mouth, therefore, liquid drenches are dangerous. A paste made from Potassi Chlorate, two ounces; Potassi Nitrate, two ounces, dissolved in a pint of warm molasses and given well back on the tongue in tablespoonful doses every two or three hours is very beneficial. A liniment made from equal parts of Aqua Ammonia Fort., Turpentine and Sweet Oil should be applied, every morning over the enlargement that appears in the region of the throat. If the enlargement fails to come to a head, secure the services of an accomplished veterinarian, who will use a clean instrument for lancing purposes.

After an attack of distemper your horse is generally run down in condition. Give the following: Potassi Nitrate, four ounces; Pulv. Gentian Root, four ounces; Pulv. Anise Seed, eight ounces. Make into thirty-two powders and give one powder three times daily in feed.

DROPSY

(Of the Belly, Chest, Sheath, Udder and Legs)

CAUSE: Poor circulation; kidneys not working properly; lack of exercise; diseases of the lungs, liver, heart, womb or sheath. Mares heavy with foal often have dropsical swellings.

SYMPTOMS: Swelling seldom contains fluid, although sometimes a sticky serum oozes through the skin; fingers pressed against the swollen parts leave impressions.

TREATMENT: Avoid giving physics in this condition when possible, especially to mares with foal. Feed laxative food, as hot bran mashes, green grass, carrots, potatoes, etc.; also the following mixture: Potassi Iodide, two ounces; Potassi Nitrate, four ounces; Chloride of Potash, two ounces. Mix and make into sixteen powders. Place one powder in their drinking water three times a day. Exercise the animal as much as possible and you will derive good results from this treatment within a week or so.

I may add that in the above affection it is a bad practice to apply hot applications, as the chances are it would produce a sloughing of the skin.

ECZEMA

CAUSE: Anything that interferes with the healthy action of the skin, as checked sweating, irritation from dirty blankets or harness, or from accumulation of dirt on the skin through want of grooming, errors in feeding, overheat, or by infection. In some cases the cause seems to be constitutional; in others, local. Though the disease is not parasitic in character, it is probable that when once contracted the diseased parts may be become infected.

SYMPTOMS: Slight dryness and eruptions that may affect the head, ears, neck, shoulders, flanks, inside of thighs and root of the tail, followed by vesicles or pimples which burst and discharge, or the contents may be absorbed. The animal will rub against the stall, manger, or any other object he can reach, until the parts are very sore, or if worked, he will rub himself violently when unharnessed.

TREATMENT: Give Fowler's Solution of Arsenic, one tablespoonful morning and night on their feed; also give a physic consisting of two drams of Aloin and two drams of Pulverized Ginger in gelatin capsule. Give at one dose. One physic is all that is necessary to cool out the blood, which will assist materially in treating Eczema. Also, apply Zinc Ointment twice daily over the vesicles or pimples which will appear on the skin. Also, feed easily digested food if possible, such as carrots, apples, grass, hot bran mashes and steamed rolled oats, and keep the animal clean and groom carefully with clean combs and brushes.

EYE DISEASES

CONJUNCTIVITIS, or Inflammation of the superficial structure of the eye.

CAUSE: Direct or indirect injury to the eye, as a blow from a whip, dust, sand or chaff in the eye, or it may be due to extreme cold, heat, or foul air.

Inflammation of the Membrane of Nictitans

The membrane of nictation is an accessory eyelid common to all domestic animals, the purpose of which is to remove foreign substances from the eye in much the same manner as we use the hand.

SYMPTOMS: Conjunctivitis and inflammation of the membranes of nictitans are very much the same. A partial or complete closure of the eye, and a watery discharge due to overstimulation of the lachrymal glands, the fluid being secreted so abundantly that it is impossible for the tear duct to carry it away; hence, there will be a continuous overflow of tears down the horse's face. The formation of a film or scum over the eye need not cause alarm if the eye shows no sign of puncture.

TREATMENT: Examine the eye carefully and remove any foreign body with clean cloth or feather and apply the following: Yellow Oxide of Mercury, three grains; Lanolin, one ounce. Mix well together and apply to the eye three or four times daily. Avoid the use of liquid medicines, as they are hard to apply, and the animal throws them out by shaking the head.

FISTULOUS WITHERS

CAUSE: Fistulous Withers are seen mostly in horses that have a thick neck as well as those that are very high in the withers, or among saddle horses, those that are very low on the withers, the saddle here riding forward and bruising the parts. They are often caused by ill-fitting collars or saddles, by direct injury from blows, and from the horse rolling upon rough, sharp stones. In this location, the ulcer of the skin or a simple abscess, if not properly and punctually treated, may terminate into Fistula. The pus burrows and finds lodgment deep down between the muscles, and escapes only when the sinuses become surcharged when, during motion of the muscles, the pus is forced to the surface.

SYMPTOMS: These of course will vary according to the progress made by the Fistula. Following an injury we may often notice soreness or stiffness of the front legs, and upon careful examination of the withers we will see small tortuous lines running from the point of irritation downwards and backwards over the region of the shoulder. The stiffness of the limbs may disappear at this time, and heat and soreness of the parts may become less noticeable, but the swelling of the shoulders continues to enlarge. The swelling may often have the form of a running ulcer, or its contents may dry up and leave a tumor, which gradually develops the common characteristic of a fistulous tumor. When the enlargement has an opening, we should carefully examine the pus cavity, as upon this condition will wholly depend our treatment.

TREATMENT: Keep the animal as quiet as possible, as any movements of the limbs cause the pus to spread between the lines of the muscles and form larger abscesses or tumors. When the bone becomes diseased, it is very difficult to effect a cure, especially where the pus burrows back of the Scapula (Shoulder Blade). In case the abscess is newly formed, and close to the surface, syringing out with a solution made from Bichloride of Mercury, five grains to one ounce of water, generally causes the white fibrous tissue to slough away and the parts to heal rapidly. If the abscess is deep, and the bones become diseased, the pus will have a very offensive odor, and I would recommend the services of a competent Veterinarian to remove all diseased portions of bone or muscle.

FILARIAE

(Thread-like Worm)

CAUSE: Drinking stagnant water, or eating hay gathered from swamps or marshy land. When full grown, the worm measures from two to six inches in length; the tail is more or less curved. They are found in the lung cavity, the heart sac, and the intestinal cavity, from which they sometimes descend into the sac containing the testicles. Animals said to have a snake in the eye have been exhibited as curiosities; in all cases the simulated snake was nothing more than the Filariae.

SYMPTOMS: Colicky spells; poor appetite, indigestion, pot-belly, rough coat; swelling of the sheath, legs, and the lower surface of the belly.

TREATMENT: Prevention is the only treatment, for when the worms once enter the digestive canal, it is impossible to remove them.

FOUNDER

CAUSE: Overeating or drinking--in fact, any irritation of the stomach or intestines is liable to be followed by Founder, owing to the similarity in the sensitive structure of the foot, skin, and mucous membranes. Horses with weak feet are predisposed to Founder, but it may also occur in strong-footed animals. Founder is also produced by driving an animal on a hot summer day and then placing in the stable where the sweat is suddenly checked by drafts, etc.

SYMPTOMS: The horse is stiff, and moves with great difficulty; he will generally, though not always, remain standing. Throws weight upon the heel of the foot to relieve the toe, and if an effort is made to back him he will drag his feet. Excessive heat is present at the top of the hoof, and a throbbing of the arteries may be felt. When the fore feet only are affected, the horse will relieve them of as much weight as possible when walking by placing the hind feet well under the body, which results in a peculiar jumping motion. Founder may occur in all four feet, but the fore feet are more often affected than the hind ones. Mares sometimes founder after giving birth to a colt, due to inflammation of the womb; symptoms correspond to those of common Founder. Founder may be mistaken for disease of the lungs or kidneys, owing to the standing position and arched back. Veterinarians have been known to mistake it for lung fever; the services of such men are dangerous and should be avoided.

TREATMENT: In all cases of Founder, administer Potassi Iodide, one ounce; Soda Bicarbonate, four ounces; Potassi Nitrate, four ounces. Mix and give one tablespoonful in drinking water every six hours. If the animal will not take it in its water, place in gelatin capsule and give with capsule gun.

Find out the true cause of the disease, if possible, and perhaps a physic will be indicated, containing Aloin, two drams; Ginger, two drams; place it in a capsule and give with capsule gun. If desired results are not obtained in eighteen hours, repeat the dose until there is an action of the bowels. Founder following excessive irritation of the stomach and intestines, or mares heavy with foal, should not receive physics. Feed food that is easily digested, as carrots, kale, apples, potatoes, hot bran mashes, or steamed rolled oats, etc.

It is well to elevate the hind quarters and give rectal injections of Warm Water and Glycerine. Stand in mud or water, or apply bags containing mud, bran or ice; in fact, anything that will have a cool, moist effect on the feet.

After the inflammation of the feet has subsided, and the animal walks fairly well, you should apply a blister containing Red Iodide of Mercury, two drams; Lard, two ounces, around the top of the hoofs, and rub in well twice forty-eight hours apart. In some cases of Founder it is recommended to bleed the animal in the foot. If this is attempted, good disinfectants should be used, as lock-jaw might follow.

GALLS

CAUSE: Injuries from ill-fitting collars, saddles, harness, hobbles and scalping-boots.

TREATMENT: Remove the cause. Never wash a Gall with water, as this prevents its healing, nor use oils or salves, as they accumulate dirt, dust and germs, which may cause infection. The following application makes a very valuable dressing for Galls: Boracic Acid, one ounce; Corn Starch, one ounce; Tannic Acid, one-half ounce; Iodoform, one dram. Powder finely and place in sifter-top can. Dust on Gall before going to work and on retiring. This heals and refreshes the Galls and wounds by forming a smooth surface over the part, which permits it to heal while the horse works.

GREASE HEEL

CAUSE: Parasitic fungi invading cracked heels.

SYMPTOMS: Offensive discharge from the glands under the skin, and if not properly treated, red spots will appear, and the yellow discharge will form a hard crust sticking to the roots of the hair.

TREATMENT: Cleanliness is one of the most important measures. Also, good nourishing food. If the skin is swollen and tender, poultice with hot Flaxseed Meal or bran. After the swelling and tenderness have abated, wash well with good Castile Soap and Warm Water. Dry with clean cloth and apply the following mixture: Calomel, one dram; Iodoform, one dram; Boracic Acid, one ounce. Mix well and apply two to three times a day. Feed green grass, carrots, kale, apples, or potatoes if possible, also feed hot bran mashes. In all cases of Grease Heel give the following physic: Aloin, two drams; Pulv. Ginger, two drams. Place in a capsule and give with capsule gun. A physic has a very good effect on the blood, which assists materially in healing the cracks and nodules that appear in Grease Heel.

GLANDERS OR FARCY

CAUSE: Due to a specific germ called the Bacillus Malleii, or Bacillus of Glanders. Glanders, or Farcy, is very contagious, and is transmissible to man as well as animals. Cattle and sheep alone are immune. The disease may be contracted at watering troughs, stables, horseshoeing shops, in boats, trains and by harness, bits, curry combs, bedding, pails, etc., as well as by direct contact with a diseased animal.

SYMPTOMS: Animal does not thrive although the appetite is good at times; loss of flesh, and is subject to sweats, the hair looks rough, the temperature increasing slightly, perhaps two degrees, a cough is generally present. Legs and abdomen are swollen; discharge from the nose, sometimes tinged with blood and very sticky, the membranes of the nose look dusty, and ulcers or spots are visible if closely examined. The glands under the back of the ears and between the jaws are hard, lumpy and swollen.

In addition to the above symptoms, Farcy affects the skin by producing swellings, or nodules, varying from the size of a pea to that of a hickory nut (called Farcy buds, or Farcy buttons), which are found inside of the hind legs under the abdomen, on the side of the chest; shoulder and neck, also around the nose, lips and face. Generally there is a discharge of greenish-yellow pus, which is very sticky.

Glanders, or Farcy, may be mistaken for nasal catarrh, nasal gleet, ulcerated teeth, nettle rash, lymphangitis, distemper, etc. Fortunately, this dreaded disease is not very prevalent in this country, as every precaution has been taken to stamp it out.

NO TREATMENT: If at any time you have reason to think one of your animals has the disease, or even a neighbor's, or a transient horse, exhibits the symptoms, it is your duty to report the fact to the State Veterinarian at once. You will do this if you have your own welfare and that of your neighborhood at heart.

HEAVES

(Emphysema of the Lungs)

CAUSE: Fast or heavy work. It may follow Lung Fever or Pleurisy, or the animal may inherit weakness in the walls of the air-cells of the lungs. A very common cause is feeding dusty or dirty hay, or bulky food. Horses that are accustomed to eating ravenously are often victims of Heaves.

SYMPTOMS: Disease may develop slowly or rapidly. When the animal is at rest, the air is taken into the lungs in a more or less normal manner, but is expelled by two distinct efforts, the abdominal muscles aiding the lungs in expiration, as may be seen by the heaving of the flank; the movement of the ribs in breathing is scarcely noticeable in a heavy horse. A healthy animal, when at rest, will throw the air from the lungs in a single effort. The difficulty in breathing is constant and increases in proportion to the amount of food in the stomach and intestines. At the beginning of the attack there is a spasmodic cough, which is more or less intermittent; this develops later into a short, weak, suppressed cough, as if the animal lacked strength in his chest to expel a full breath, often accompanied by expulsion of wind from the anus, which is somewhat protruded.

TREATMENT: Feed good, nourishing food, but nothing that is of a bulky nature. Feed more grain and less hay, which should be dampened with water if dusty. Do not feed dusty, musty or bulky food, but give plenty of potatoes, apples, kale and green grass. Have your druggist make you up one quart of Fowler's Solution of Arsenic, omitting the Tincture of Lavender. This is soothing to the organs of breathing, and should be given two tablespoonfuls three times a day on the feed. After a week or ten days you might increase the dose slightly. Although this will make the horse work much better, do not give it with the hope of effecting a complete cure, as very few cases recover fully from this disease.

HORSE DENTISTRY

This is a very important branch of Veterinary Science, although, if I were to go into detail on the subject, it would require the writing of an individual volume. This science requires considerable practice. The price of special costly instruments would prohibit the average stockman from doing his own dentistry.

My advice is to secure nothing but the services of a qualified Veterinarian, who has had privileges of a thorough knowledge of Veterinary Science.

The art of animal dentistry has been abused by the owners of stock allowing the services of irresponsible men in the veterinary profession, who do not look to the betterment of the animal's condition. The owner of the animal, not being able to see the condition of the animal's teeth for himself, is persuaded into having the animal's teeth worked on regardless of whether it is needed or not. The quack or transient Veterinarian will pull and crack healthy, sound teeth, and also lacerate the poor animal's mouth. Be sure the Veterinarian employed for this purpose is competent.

INFLUENZA

(Pink Eye-Epizootic Catarrh)

CAUSE: Influenza is a specific and infectious fever, which shows a marked tendency to rapidly spread over a large area of country. It generally appears suddenly, without, preliminary symptoms, and may become fully developed in twenty-four hours.

SYMPTOMS: The usual symptoms are those of Catarrh, although the bowels, lungs and brain complications may be present, either singly or combined. It always gives rise to great weakness. The distinguishing characteristics of Influenza from Distemper, Sore Throat, and other diseases affecting the organs of breathing, are the suddenness of the attack, rise of temperature, varying from 103 to 106 degrees F., pulse feeble and fast, and a pinkish, swollen appearance of the inside of the eyelids. The animal is dull, in some cases almost unconscious. Sometimes the legs are very stiff and swollen, and there is great difficulty in moving about.

TREATMENT: Place the affected animal in a clean, well ventilated stall, avoid drafts, give pure water to drink with chill taken off, in small quantities but often. Blanket if the weather is chilly, hand rub the legs and bandage, give Quinine, two drams, in a gelatin capsule with capsule gun every four hours. In addition to the above, administer the treatment recommended for Acute and Chronic Coughs.

Feed good, nutritious food that has a laxative effect on the bowels, as it is dangerous to give horses physic with this disease. Hot bran mashes, steamed rolled oats and vegetables are very beneficial.

LAMPAS

CAUSE: In young horses it is commonly caused by cutting teeth. In older animals it is usually due to indigestion.

SYMPTOMS: A puffy swelling and redness of the gums. The animal may have difficulty in eating.

TREATMENT: In young animals, when cutting teeth, let nature take its course, but when an animal is five years or over, place two drams of Aloin, and two drams of Pulv. Ginger, in a gelatin capsule and administer with capsule gun. Then tone up the digestive organs by mixing one ounce of Pulv. Gentian Root, one ounce of Pulv. Nux Vomica, four ounces of Bicarbonate of Soda. Make into eight powders and give one powder in feed twice daily, or place in gelatin capsule and administer with capsule gun.

LEECHES

(Haemopis)

The leeches which suck the blood of the horse may be divided into two classes, the external parasites which attach themselves to the skin of the legs and adjacent parts of the horse, and the Haemopis Sanguisuga, and others of this class, which, not being able to penetrate the skin, endeavor to enter the mouth or nostrils of the horse when he is drinking or grazing in wet and leech-infected pastures. They sometimes cling to the mucous membrane of the eyes. The horse leech, which lives in the water, usually gains access to the mouth and nostrils of the animal, when young and not more than one-tenth of an inch long. They rarely go beyond the air and food passages, generally fastening themselves to the walls of the windpipe and gullet, where they cling till the animal dies from loss of blood or suffocation. They often cause bleeding from the mouth and nostrils, and may be seen by close examination.

TREATMENT: Endeavor to build up the condition of the animal with suitable food. Also feed liberal quantities of stock salt. Where the leeches cling tightly to the mucous membranes of the mouth and nostrils, it is well to cause the horse to inhale the vapor from hot water containing turpentine.

LOCK-JAW

(Tetanus)

CAUSE: The bacilli of Tetanus are widely distributed and can be found in practically every part of the globe. Their favorite place of production, however, is in barn yards and marshy ground. They are frequently swallowed by stock along with forage, and can often be found in recently expelled feces. The most favorable temperature for their development is about 70 degrees F. They act by means of extremely virulent poisons which they produce, and which causes the terrible symptoms that are characteristic of the disease.

SYMPTOMS: The muscles of expression are usually the first brought under the continual spasm of tetanus, and when thus affected give the face of the animal a pinched and drawn-in appearance. The other muscles of the head and those of the neck are next attacked. The mouth is closed, the nose poked out, the head elevated. The muscles of breathing, and those of the limbs, become contracted so that the neck is hollowed, and the tail is raised, the horse stands with outstretched limbs. The animal shows great stiffness or rigidity in attempted movements. The eyes are sunken, and when startled or excited, the breathing is quickened and the flanks have a wrinkled or corrugated appearance. Death may quickly occur from continuous spasms of the muscles of the throat. Another sign is the flying up of the accessory eyelid when the animal is excited.

TREATMENT: If noticed in its first stages, and if the animal is able to eat, secure the services of an accomplished Veterinarian and insist on the use of fresh vaccine. This disease is almost impossible to cure, and about ninety per cent die.

LUNG FEVER

(Pneumonia)

CAUSE: Predisposition is largely accountable for this disease, which is more common to young horses than old; also, changes of temperature, introduction of foreign bodies or liquids into the trachea (windpipe) and the bronchial tubes, inhalation of smoke or irritating gases, excitement, exposure to cold after clipping, turning out to pasture from a warm stable, or injury to chest or ribs from being struck with a pole, etc.

SYMPTOMS: Dullness in spirit; animal usually shivers or trembles; when this ceases the temperature rises to perhaps 103 to 106 degrees F., pulse increases to sixty or ninety per minute, full and bounding; breathing short and labored and abnormally quick, increasing to perhaps fifty inspirations per minute, whereas in health it does not exceed twelve or thirteen per minute. A cough is also likely to be present, and the animals remain standing until they are on the road to recovery, or until death takes place. Other symptoms are constipation, feces covered with mucus or slime; urination frequent, scanty and dark in color; appetite poor, but thirst great; the eyes look glassy and the membranes have an inflamed appearance. It is a good sign if the animal looks about freely. When the critical stage is past the temperature and pulse gradually fall, the appetite returns and the urine becomes more abundant, and takes on its natural color, the cough loosens, and the discharge from the lungs is profuse, and of a yellowish color, and the breathing becomes normal.

TREATMENT: Good care is of the utmost importance. Place the horse in a comfortable, well ventilated stall, being careful to exclude drafts. Hand rub and bandage the legs with woolen cloth. Blanket the animal, give plenty of bedding and keep pure water before him at all times. Internally administer Quinine, two ounces; Iodide of Ammonia, two ounces; Ammonia Bicarbonate, two ounces. Mix well and make into sixteen powders. Place powder in gelatin capsule and give with capsule gun every four hours. It is quite necessary that the above remedy should be placed in capsule, as drugs of this nature tend to irritate the throat. Do not give physics, as it is much safer to give laxative food, as hot bran mashes, steam rolled oats or some vegetables, in fact anything the animal will eat, i.e., that has food values. It is advisable to apply over the chest the following liniment; Aqua Ammonia Fort., four ounces; Turpentine, four ounces; Raw Linseed Oil, four ounces. Mix and shake well before applying each time over the chest cavity.

In case the animal is constipated, give rectal injections of soap and warm water containing a few drops of Turpentine.

MANGE

(Scabies)

CAUSE: Mange is a contagious disease, produced by the presence of a small parasite that varies in length from a fiftieth to a hundredth of an inch, according to the species, of which there are three: Sarcoptes, which generally affects the withers; Symbiotes Communis, affecting the legs, and the Psoroptes Communis, which affects horses about the root of the tail and mane. The latter is the one most commonly found affecting horses. They multiply rapidly and are spread from diseased to healthy horses by their bodies coming in contact with one another, or by corrals, stables, railroad cars, etc., recently occupied by mangy horses.

SYMPTOMS: The mange mite attacks the skin and produces a thickness of its outer surface, covering it with crusts and scabs, with a consequent loss of hair. Intense itching accompanies the disease, and affected horses continually bite and rub themselves.

Psoroptic Mange commences at the root of the tail, or at the roots of the mane on the neck or withers, and gradually spreads over the back, up to the head, over the sides, and finally affects the entire body. In cases of long standing the skin becomes ulcerated, the animal becomes greatly weakened, emaciated and finally dies.

TREATMENT: When a large number of horses are affected (in one locality) it is best to prepare a vat and dip them, under the supervision of the United States Bureau of Animal Industry. When just a few horses become affected, the following has proven very effective: Sulphur, eight ounces; Oil of Tar, eight ounces; Sweet Oil, two quarts. Mix and apply liberally to the parts affected. A few applications are generally sufficient to eradicate the disease.

MONDAY MORNING DISEASE

(Lymphangitis)

CAUSE: This ailment is common with hard working horses, and is caused by confining them in the stable and allowing their usual amount of food. More nutriment is consumed than can be taken up by the system, which causes an irritation. It is frequently found in certain stables on Monday morning, hence its name--Monday Morning Disease.

SYMPTOMS: Swelling and lameness, most usually affecting the hind leg inside of the thigh and extending down the leg in a hard ridge. It will pit on pressure, and cause intense pain; the horse will have difficulty in extending the limb forward, the swelling may surround the leg entirely. Pulse will be fifty to sixty per minute, temperature 102 to 104 degrees F., breathing will be faster than normal. The animal has great thirst, but the appetite is very poor; usually remains standing; if he lies down will have great difficulty in getting up.

TREATMENT: In this particular disease apply hot fomentations to the affected limb or limbs, for one hour, then rub dry and apply Camphorated Liniment. Give Nitrate Potassi, Chlorate of Potassi, Iodide Potassi, each four ounces. Mix and make into thirty-two powders. Give one powder three times a day in drinking water or in a gelatin capsule and give with capsule gun.

In most cases it is advisable to give a physic: Aloin, two drams; Pulv. Gentian Root, one dram; Ginger, one dram. Place in gelatin capsule and give with capsule gun.

MUD FEVER

CAUSE: Horses driven over muddy roads during the day and exposed to freezing weather at night, or driving them over muddy roads, then washing the limbs and not drying them properly, often produces a superficial inflammation of the legs.

SYMPTOMS: The legs are swollen, extremely hot and tender, the horse is stiff, the hair comes off the legs easily and if the cause is not removed severe complication may follow, as the secretions of the skin become greatly affected.

TREATMENT: Prevention. Horses that are driven over muddy, wet roads should have their legs rubbed dry when stabling them for any length of time. When the legs are badly swollen wash them with clean warm water and

Castile soap and dry them well with a clean soft cloth. Then apply Zinc Oxide Ointment or a lotion made from Acetate of Lead, one ounce; Zinc Sulphate, one-half ounce. Place in a quart of clean water and apply twice daily. Either application is very beneficial in the treatment of Mud Fever. Feed the animal wheat bran mashes, steamed rolled oats, vegetables, etc., as they have a very good effect on the system which aids in relieving the inflammation of the skin.

NASAL GLEET

(Chronic Catarrh)

CAUSE: Exposure to cold followed by neglect, and lack of nourishing food; bruise or fracture of the frontal bones of the head; injury of the blood-vessels inside the bones, or an ulcerated tooth. May also be caused by tumor, or foreign substance or liquids in the nasal cavities. Sometimes dried pus in the nostrils, resulting from a cold, will cause nasal gleet.

SYMPTOMS: A white or yellowish discharge from one or both of the nostrils, the quantity varying with the severity of the attack and the length of time the disease has been established. If, when tapping over the nose below the eye, a dull sound is produced, it is safe to conclude that the cavities are filled with pus; to make certain, compare the sick animal with a healthy one; in some cases you will notice that even the bones of the nose below the eye are slightly elevated. The lining of the nose may be of a red or yellow color but not ulcerated in spots, as in Glanders. The animal may continue in pretty good spirits and work well for a time but as the case develops he becomes lean in flesh and what is termed hide-bound. Always examine the teeth. In a case of long standing, the discharge has a fetid smell, differing in this respect also from Glanders.

TREATMENT: If not due to fractured bones of the head or ulcerated teeth, the animal will, in most cases, recover with proper medical treatment. When due to injury to the bones of the head, tumors, ulcerated teeth or dried pus in the nasal cavities, it is best to secure the services of a skillful Veterinarian, one whose professional knowledge renders him thoroughly competent. In the mild forms of nasal-gleet or chronic catarrh, administer the following: Ferri Sulphate, Potassi Iodide, Nux Vomica, each four ounces. Mix well and make into thirty-two capsules. Give one capsule three times daily and feed food that is nourishing and easily digested.

NAVEL STRING INFECTION

(Umbilical Pyemia)

CAUSE AND NATURE: While the unborn foal (foetus) is in the womb of its mother, it is surrounded by enveloping membranes which constitute the after-birth on delivery. These membranes are attached to the wall of the womb and are connected to the foetus by means of the navel-string (umbilical cord) which is provided with two arteries and a vein for the nourishment of the young creature and for the removal of its waste products.

It also has a narrow canal (the urachus) which serves to remove the urine of the foetus; in fact the subsequently formed bladder takes its origin from a dilation of the urachus. Under normal conditions when the foal is born, respiration takes place, the umbilical arteries and veins become quickly blocked up, urine is discharged through the urethra (which communicates with the penis or vagina, as the case may be), the foal enjoys a separate existence and the wound caused by the division of the umbilical cord leaves a scar which is known as the navel.

It is usually supposed that the germ of navel-string infection gains admittance into the body through the exposed surface before the wound is closed. However, I am of the opinion that the mother is the bearer of the infection in a great many cases for in the uterine secretions of mares whose foals fell with navel-string infection, the same characteristic germs were found as were present in the joints of the affected foals. The infectious material is, by the act of covering, conveyed from mare to mare, so that the mucous membranes of the womb becomes the habitat of the specific germ. By inoculation of these germs into the blood stream of foals an illness is produced which in the smallest particular cannot be distinguished from that arising in naturally affected foals. It is a strange fact that when the infected germs are transmitted by the mother, their presence does not produce any disturbance in her.

This is a very common malady in most places. I have known several instances on particular farms where they were unable to raise either foals or calves, but if the mother were removed to another farm immediately after or before foaling, the foal or calf lived and was reared without difficulty, and although constitutional debility plays an important part, the presence of specific germs constituting an infected area is, I believe, the most important factor in producing this disease.

According to my observation, about seventy-five per cent of the cases die within the first three weeks after birth. This high rate of mortality would be considerably diminished if proper treatment was adopted.

SYMPTOMS: The attack usually comes on during the second or third week after birth and almost always before the closure of the navel opening, which, in affected animals, will be found to be in a wet and suppurating condition. Occasionally foals two or three months old which have the urachus closed and are in an apparently healthy condition contract this disease in a form of painful swelling of the joints. The first symptoms are generally dullness; more or less fever; lameness which is often attributed to rheumatism or to injury caused by the mare treading on the foal; the disinclination to move or even to stand. Upon examination the patient will be found to have a soft, gelatinous swelling of one or more of the joints of which the hock, elbow, fetlock, stifle and hip usually manifest the enlargement most clearly.

These swellings are hot and painful to the touch; they tend to suppurate and frequently cause intense lameness. In very rare cases open urachus may exist without any joint inflammation. In this disease, inflammation of the joints and open urachus are almost always co-existent.

Animals that recover from a bad attack are seldom worth the trouble of rearing, because as a rule their constitution becomes permanently impaired and one or more of their joints becomes stiffened by the attack.

TREATMENT: In the treatment of this disease, we have to attend to constitutional disturbances, inflamed joints, open urachus and complications such as constipation and diarrhoea. The comfort of our little patient must be studied under all circumstances. If the weather be at all cold it should be covered by a warm sheet. Should the foal have any difficulty in rising from the recumbent position, an attendant should assist it to rise and see that it is regularly fed. It is only in extreme cases that the animal refuses to suck its dam. During warm weather, and especially if the ground is dry, such a patient is always better off for a little sunshine, but on no account must it be left out during extreme heat, as in this state it is very liable to sunstroke. The best food for the mare is grass, which, during the day, she can generally have. The inflamed joints of the foal should be rubbed lightly with the following, after being thoroughly mixed: Red Iodide of Mercury, two drams; Vaseline, two ounces, every forty-eight hours, which, when applied to the skin, appears to have a well-marked antiseptic action on the underlying tissues. An inflamed joint should on no account be bathed with warm water, fomented or poulticed because the application of moist heat would be the best possible means for promoting the development of the infective germs which are the cause of the local and general disturbance. The open navel-string should not be ligatured because that operation is generally followed by an increased inflammation of the part, and by an aggravation of the other symptoms apparently on account of this outlet for deleterious products becoming blocked up. If the navel-string has been ligatured and is in an inflamed state, the ligature should be removed without delay. If the foal is constipated give two to three ounces of Castor Oil; also, administer the following: Zinc Sulphocarbolates, one-half dram; Hyposulphite of Soda, four ounces. Mix and make into thirty-two powders. Give one powder well back on the tongue every four hours.

As a supplement to the food, we may give brown sugar or treacle, both of which are easily digested and are very nourishing. Four or five eggs daily will also aid in keeping up the strength.

NAVEL RUPTURE

(Umbilical Hernia)

CAUSE: Hereditary predisposition is well marked in this complaint. It may exist at birth, but so-called congenital rupture may very probably be the result of the pulling which the navel-string underwent at the time of foaling. However, umbilical hernia usually occurs during the first two or three months after birth; that is to say, while the opening at the navel is becoming obliterated and the tissues at that place are becoming consolidated. They can, however, appear later and may result from more or less violent strains sustained when the foals are jumping or playing. At other times these strains are induced by intestinal irritation accompanied by diarrhoea or constipation with straining. But, however the strain may take place, the abdominal muscles contract and push the intestines towards the wall of the belly. Then if they find an opening or even a weak spot, like the ring of the navel while it is undergoing the process of becoming blocked up, they select it and a rupture is produced.

SYMPTOMS: This rupture, the situation of which clearly shows its character, may vary in size from that of a hen's egg to that of an ostrich's egg. If pressed upon with the hand, especially if the animal is placed on its back, the rupture will disappear, to return, however, when the pressure is removed. If it be composed of intestines it will be soft and elastic when the bowels are empty, but when they are full of semi-solid food they will be doughy. In any event, the tumor will feel elastic when composed of intestines, but when formed of its connecting membranes, will naturally not vary in consistence. If intestines be present, movements and abdominal rumblings may be detected in it. This rupture rarely gives rise to serious consequences because its contents are composed of large intestines and omentum, either of which is, in this position, not liable to become strangulated. It may, however, become engorged and inflamed from injury. Its existence naturally depreciates the value of an animal suffering from it.

TREATMENT: In the majority of cases, they will disappear with their own accord in two or three months. In case the rupture shows no signs of diminishing in size it is well to apply a bandage around the abdomen or secure the services of a competent veterinarian and he will prescribe a treatment or operate, which will apply directly to your colt's or horse's particular case.

OPEN JOINT

CAUSE: Injuries such as a kick from a sharp shoe, wire cuts, punctures from snags, or from probing a wound near a joint. Open joint is one of the most serious accidents that may happen to a horse, for the sufferer is apt to die from the ensuing constitutional disturbance, and even if he recovers the joint will, in all probability, be permanently stiff.

SYMPTOMS: If the joint is opened or severely injured the wound will have an ordinary appearance except that there may be a flow of joint oil from the injured oil sack. However, the discharge gradually becomes more unhealthy until finally it is mixed with pus and blood and assumes a fetid odor. After two or three days the joint swells and becomes very painful and a high fever sets in. In unfavorable cases the animal dies from exhaustion very shortly, or at best recovers with a permanently stiff joint.

TREATMENT: Never probe a wound near a joint. If the injury is small and noticed immediately, apply Red Iodide of Mercury, two drams; Vaseline, two ounces. Mix and rub in well over the wound. This will set up sufficient inflammation to close the opening and kill any infection that may be present, as it possesses powerful antiseptic properties. If the wound is large, wash with Bichloride of Mercury, one part to one thousand parts distilled water. The wound should be washed twice a day with this solution. Then dust the wound with Tannic Acid, one ounce; Iodoform, one ounce; Boracic Acid, one ounce; Calomel, one dram. Mix and place in sifter top can and apply this after washing each time. Then bandage the wound by first placing clean absorbent cotton over the wound. Do not attempt to syringe a solution into an opening or some of the solution may gain entrance into the joint. Keep the animal as quiet as possible and feed laxative food.

PALESADE WORM

(Strongulus Armatus)

This parasite thrives on marshy ground and is commonly found in the United States and Canada. The body of the worm is gray in color, more or less stiff and straight and thicker in the front than in the hind part; it varies in length, the male measuring from three-fourths of an inch to one inch and the female from one to two inches. It may occur in an adult or an immature state. In the former it implants itself on the mucous membrane of the large intestines by means of its armed mouth, while in the latter it lives in cysts underneath the mucous membrane of the intestines and is sometimes found in the brain, testicles and liver. The immature worms which do not issue directly from the cysts get into the arteries and are carried by the force of the blood to all parts of the body.

SYMPTOMS: Same as in Red Worm with the exception of colicky pains caused by the worms blocking the arteries which carry blood to the intestines, thus interfering with the process of digestion. Where the worms enter the arteries of the limbs it results in lameness. It is a good plan to examine your animals once or twice a year to insure them against this pest.

TREATMENT: Same as for Red Worm.

PLEURISY

CAUSE: Exposed to a sudden change of temperature, confinement in ill-ventilated, damp stables, wounds penetrating the chest, fractured ribs, heart diseases. It also occurs in conjunction with Bronchitis, Influenza, etc.

SYMPTOMS: Generally only one side of the lungs is affected and that being the right, although it may affect both sides at the same time. First you will notice the animal distressed, uneasy, shivering, the affected side is painful to pressure of the hand. The breathing is short and quick, and the flanks heave-- which shows that the animal tries to breathe as much as possible, by the action of the muscles of the abdomen and not by the movement of the ribs. The nostrils are dilated. There is usually a short, dry, painful cough present, which is repressed by the animal as much as possible, so as not to shake the inflamed parts. Often when expelling air from the lungs the horse gives a painful grunt especially when made to move. The pulse is generally hard and faster than usual. The temperature in early stages may rise from 104 to 106 degrees F. If the ear is applied to the affected side a dry crackling or friction sound can be heard; a groove along the lower portion of the ribs will extend back to the flank. Within two or three days the pulse will be softer and weaker, temperature will fall to 101 or 102 degrees F. and there will be fluids form and the painful short breathing will disappear. The liquids may now undergo absorption if properly treated, and the case terminate favorably in a week or ten days.

Frequently large quantities of fluid accumulate in the chest cavity that cannot be absorbed, the breathing becomes more difficult, short and quick, pulse becomes weak and rapid and the animal dies from exhaustion.

TREATMENT: Place the animal in a comfortable, roomy stall; blanket if the weather is chilly, permit fresh air, but no drafts, as this is very important.

Apply a paste made from Mustard and cold water over the chest cavity. Internally, administer Ammonium Iodide, Chlorate of Potash, Nitrate of Potash, each four ounces. Make into thirty-two powders and give one powder every two or three hours in gelatin capsule and administer with capsule gun. The diet is a proper means of keeping up the animal and is very important. Coax the animal to eat grass or vegetables, hot bran mashes or steam rolled oats. If there is a cough present, give the same treatment as recommended for Acute and Chronic Coughs.

PIN WORM, THREAD OR MAW WORM

(Oxyuris Curvilis)

This worm when full grown is about one and three-quarter inches in length; its tail is thin and whip-like and head thick and terminating in a curve somewhat resembling the crook of a stick. The presence of these parasites may be detected by a light-yellow substance (the eggs of the worms) which adheres to the skin below the anus. Pin Worms like Round Worms frequently come away with the feces.

TREATMENT: Dissolve four tablespoonfuls Common Salt in one gallon of warm water and inject it into the rectum. When this has been expelled, follow with an injection per rectum of Turpentine, four ounces, to one-half gallon Linseed Oil. Elevate the horse's hind quarters so as to retain the injection longer. This will expel the worms and their eggs that cling to the walls of the rectum. The worms sometimes make their way so far forward that it is impossible to reach them with an injection. In this case treat same as for Round worms.

Where there is irritation produced about the tail the horse continually rubs and it is well to apply Mercurial Ointment to both tail and the anus.

POLL EVIL

Poll Evil is so-called because it occurs in the region of the poll. It is not a constitutional disease, but comes, no doubt, from well marked causes, as from inflammation set up and involving the bones and muscles in the region of the poll, and perhaps of the larger ligament. Owing to the low vitality of the parts and the action of the head in taking food, etc., the pus is apt to burrow deep into the muscles.

CAUSE: Direct or Indirect injury. A common cause is striking the head against a low doorway or an ill-fitting halter or bridle.

SYMPTOMS: Swelling just back of the ears on one or both sides of the head. The animal stands with the nose out; slight heat in the parts, pain on pressure. In the first stages, it is merely inflammatory action. The second stage is suppuration, or there may be great swelling in some cases when there is but little pus formed.

In other cases there is profuse suppuration and the pus makes its way out and discharges to the surface and sinuses are formed, which extend in various directions. Any abscess in this region is called Poll Evil.

TREATMENT: When the enlargement is first noticed in the region of the poll, I would advise the following: Red Iodide of Mercury, four drams; Lard, four ounces, rub in well over the enlargement and perhaps this will prevent sinuses from forming, but when the cases are long standing and so-called pipes are formed, I would advise that you secure the services of an accomplished Veterinarian.

PETECHIAL FEVER

(Purpura Haemorrhagica)

CAUSE: Constitutional weakness following some debilitating disease such as Distemper, Pink Eye, Catarrh and even following operations, when an animal becomes weak and from want of exercise, in which case it generally appears during his recovery. It is not infectious and cannot be transmitted by inoculations.

SYMPTOMS: There is a slight swelling of the limbs, more likely to be about the hocks. The swelling may disappear by exercising, but will soon return. The swellings present a very abrupt appearance, nearly the same as if a string were tied around the limbs and swell very quickly, and symptomatic of Purpura. Exudations take place in which, if on white limbs, you will see little red spots, from which a liquid is oozing. The swelling is very painful and the entire limb may be swollen. Small vesicles appear on the limbs and also in the mucous membranes, and it is well to look at the mucous membranes before giving your opinion, as you will, no doubt, detect these spots, which may extend into the lungs. These spots increase and may run into each other. The mucous membranes of the nose may become a mass of corrupt matter. The upper lip may hang pendulous, which is due to the want of nervous stimulus. If the nostrils are swollen very badly, there is difficulty in breathing and if the animal is not able to take food, the symptoms are considered very bad. The pulse varies much in some cases; although the swelling is very great, the pulse may not be more than forty or fifty per minute. The temperature is elevated one to three degrees above normal, there may be a coughing and a brownish colored discharge from the nostrils. The mouth and eyes become affected and, together with the discharge from the nose, the horse is a loathsome looking object. In milder cases the appetite is retained, or the animal may take food one day and the next refuse it. The bowels are constipated as a general thing in the first stages of the disease and the urine may be of a dark color, may even contain blood. There may be a peculiar dropsical swelling of these petechial spots or it may show itself in connection with the eyes and there may be blood extravasation without outer symptoms. This disease may affect the bowels, liver, lungs, etc. The animal usually stands, perhaps from the difficulty in moving the limbs. It is necessary to watch the case closely for flies will attack him and he will be filled with maggots. Sloughing may take place; the entire sheath or patches upon the body may slough off and there may be paralysis of the penis.

TREATMENT: Place the animal in a clean, light, comfortable stall. If the weather is cold, blanket. The following medicine is recommended because of its particular effect on the blood in this disease: Chlorate of Potash, eight ounces; Iodide of Potash, eight ounces; Quinine Sulphate, eight ounces. Make into thirty-two capsules and give one capsule every six hours. Also administer one ounce capsules filled with Spirits of Turpentine three or four times a day. Moisten the capsules with Sweet Oil and give with capsule gun. Feed hot bran mashes containing two or three ounces of pure Flaxseed meal. Also, feed vegetables, green grass, if possible.

QUITTOR

(Fistula of the Foot)

CAUSE: Injuries. Horses working on rough stony roads are subject to punctures, pricks, bruises, corns, treads, etc., which end in pus formation which does not get a pendant opening and destroys the tissues with which it comes in contact. Finally it bursts, forms sinuses and pipes, as commonly called, at the top of the hoof.

SYMPTOMS: Extreme lameness, heat, pain and swelling will show themselves about the top of the hoof. As a rule a Quittor develops slowly and is more or less painful during the first stages. After the sinus is formed and the pus discharges, the inflammation generally subsides. Its healing process is often delayed due to the diseased portion of the cartilages inside the horny hoof.

TREATMENT: Apply Flaxseed or hot Bran poultices to relieve the inflammation and hasten the formation of sinuses or pipes. Then with an ordinary syringe inject the following: Silver Nitrate, ten grains; Water, one ounce. Inject fifteen to twenty drops twice daily. Keep the food clean and the animal as quiet as possible. It is very disagreeable, as stated before, and the healing is very slow, but this must be naturally expected, as we are unable to provide the sinuses with good drainage.

RED WORM

(Strongylus Tetracanthus)

The Red Worm varies in length from one-third to three and one-quarter inches, and is sometimes white though it usually appears to be red because of the blood it contains. This parasite is found in all parts of the world. Its favorite haunt is marshy land.

SYMPTOMS: Paleness of all visible membranes, eyes watery and inflamed, swelling of the sheath, legs, and lower surface of the belly; fetid diarrhoea, dullness, debility, emaciation, rough coat, and the presence of worms in the feces. The worms when first passed are bright red in color but after being exposed to the air they turn dark and may easily escape the notice of the casual observer.

TREATMENT: Withhold all food for twenty-four hours, then place the following drugs in a gelatin capsule: Calomel, two drams, Barbadoes Aloes, three drams; Ferri Sulphate, two drams. Give with capsule gun. Also place the following tonic in their feed: Pulv. Quassia, one ounce; Ferri Sulphate, two ounces; Pulv. Anise Seed, two ounces. Mix and make sixteen powders. Give one powder two or three times a day in the feed.

RHEUMATISM

CAUSE: Exposure to cold rains, drafts, lying on damp ground when the blood is in poor condition. Also due to over-stimulating food.

SYMPTOMS: Lameness, swelling or soreness which may shift from one place to another, then finally locate in or near one of the joints of the limbs.

TREATMENT: Take away all grains and feed laxative foods such as potatoes, carrots, apples, kale and good hay. If the weather is warm turn out to pasture, but confine in warm stable at night. It is advisable to give a physic, as Aloin, two drams; Gentian, one dram; Ginger, one dram. Place in gelatin capsule and give at one dose with capsule gun, as its action on the blood has a very good effect. When the swellings are painful, apply Camphorated Liniment once or twice daily. Also, administer the following tonic: Potassi Iodide, one ounce; Nitrate of Potash, two ounces; Chlorate of Potash, two ounces; Pulv. Gentian Root, one ounce; Ferri Sulphate, one ounce; Pulv. Anise Seed, four ounces. Mix well and make into twenty powders. Give one powder three times a day in bran or place in capsule and give with capsule gun.

RING BONE

CAUSE: Faulty conformation--as a narrow or straight pastern joint is considered faulty. Be very careful in selecting a sire when breeding, as faulty conformation is hereditary. Ringbone may also result when young animals are put to work on hard roads or running in stony pastures sometimes produces Ringbone before the bones have become properly hardened. Other causes are injury to tendons or ligaments, bruised joints, blows, calking, or picking up a nail.

SYMPTOMS: Lameness will manifest itself when the horse first starts out in the morning; this may become less noticeable or even disappear temporarily as the animal works. They gradually grow lamer and examination will disclose an enlargement at or around the top of the hoof. This may appear in one or more feet, but the front feet are more often affected.

TREATMENT: If the Ringbone is very much inflamed, reduce the heat by applying cold water or ice packs to the part. Clip off all hair from around the top of the hoof and rub in well for twenty minutes the following: Red Iodide of Mercury, two drams; Pulv. Cantharides, two drams; Turpentine, one dram; Pine Tar, two drams, and mix in two ounces of Lard. This applied every two days for a week and repeat same treatment in two weeks. Keep the animal as quiet as possible as it assists in producing a recovery. If the animal is comparatively young, recovery is certain, although the enlargement may never disappear.

ROUND WORM

(Ascaris Megalcephala)

Resembles the Earth Worm somewhat in shape, yellowish-white in color, stiff and elastic. When full grown, it varies in length from six to sixteen inches. These worms are usually found in the small intestines, although they sometimes invade the stomach, and when numerous seriously disturb the animal's health.

SYMPTOMS: The animal's general health is affected as is evident from the morbid state of his appetite, rough coat, pot-belly, liability to colic and slight diarrhoea. Some of these worms are often expelled with the feces. As they increase in number, they block up the small intestines, giving rise to colic, and may in time kill the horse. They sometimes cause perforation of the bowels.

TREATMENT: Withhold all food from eighteen to twenty-four hours, then administer the following: Ferri Sulphate, two drams; Antimony Tartrate, two drams; Pulv. Quassia, two drams. Place in gelatin capsule and give with capsule gun. Follow this from six to eight hours with Aloin, two drams; Ginger, two drams, and give as above directed. It is a good plan to repeat the above treatment in ten days to insure the removal of any worms which may have survived the first treatment.

SCROTAL RUPTURE

(Inguinal Hernia)

CAUSE: Abnormal size of the upper ring through which a part of the intestines or its connecting membrane descends into and through the canal leading from the abdomen to the scrotal cavity. There is little danger of strangulation from this form of rupture which may occur at birth and disappear with age. A careful examination should therefore be made of the scrotum before castration.

SYMPTOMS: In most cases, this condition is easily detected. The scrotum will be somewhat enlarged. Sometimes the intestines will become strangulated and colicky symptoms appear. When a young male colt shows signs of colic, examine him for Scrotal Rupture.

TREATMENT: The trouble usually disappears with age although in some cases it is well to operate. Where colicky symptoms are present, roll the colt on its back, manipulating the scrotum. Diet carefully.

SHOE BOIL

(Capped Elbow)

CAUSE: Injuries, bruises or pressure when lying on a rough floor. Sharp heeled shoes and kicks also have a tendency to produce it.

SYMPTOMS: A hot painful swelling of the Elbow joint when first noticed. When neglected, it takes on a white fibrous or callous growth.

TREATMENT: First remove the cause. Do not lance the enlargement; let it come to a head of its own accord, by applying Red Iodide of Mercury, two drams; Pulv. Cantharides, three drams; Lard, two ounces. Mix well together and apply twice a week. When the swelling is hot and painful it is well to apply cold water or ice packs before applying the above mentioned prescription.

SPLINTS

CAUSE: This disease is chiefly produced by trotting or running on hard ground, etc. It is evident that horses with high knee action and heavy bodies are more liable to this disease. Jumping is also a common cause of splints, but the more accustomed a horse is to jumping the less liable he is to throw splints, because practice teaches the animal to regulate his movements so as to more or less diminish the disagreeable if not actually painful effect of concussion.

SYMPTOMS: A splint is detected by grasping the horse's leg with the fingers upon one side and the thumb upon the other, and tracing the inner and outer splint bones from their heads downward to their tapering extremities. Any actual enlargement will at once arrest the hand; any rising or irregularity will create suspicion and lead to close examination. Horses, especially young ones which have lately been put to work, not infrequently develop splints before any swelling appears. For this reason, in examining a case of obscure lameness, particularly if the animal is young, do not fail to look for the sign of splint lameness, namely: that the lameness is abnormally greater at a trot than at a walk and that the animal usually fails to bend the knees freely and grows worse with exercise. The last mentioned condition is also present with corns, but an examination of the foot will determine the question of their existence. In young horses splints are sometimes mistaken for coffin-joint lameness or navicular disease. To avoid this error, it should be remembered that, when brought on by navicular disease, the action of the limb improves with exercise; also that horses of five years of age or less very rarely suffer from coffin-joint disease. Some horses, owing to unusual development of the inner splint bones of the fore legs may appear to have splints, although careful examination may prove both limbs to be free from any bony deposit. When deciding such a point, note if the two inner splint bones are of the same size. Any swelling perceptible in a limb recently affected with splint-lameness is usually attended by heat and pain.

TREATMENT: If there is heat present, foment with hot or cold water; when heat has subsided, apply the following ointment: Red Iodide of Mercury, two drams; Turpentine, twenty drops, and mix. Apply every forty-eight hours until three applications have been applied. Rub in for twenty minutes each time.

During this treatment use the horse for slow work on soft roads, etc. As a rule the splints will not disappear at once, but will gradually. I may add that common splints are not considered an unsoundness.

SPASMODIC COLIC

CAUSE: Horses seem to be predisposed to this form of colic on account of the great length of their intestines which are apt to be telescoped, twisted or their circular muscular fibers spasmodically contracted. Perhaps the principal cause is a change of food, sudden change of temperature, constipation, drinking cold or too large a quantity of water, especially if the animal is warm; overloading the stomach with frozen or mouldy food. Worms frequently produce colic.

SYMPTOMS: If the animal is tied it will become uneasy, paw, point its nose to the flank, twitch the tail, lie down and get up frequently. If the animal is loose it will walk around, paw, kick at its belly with the hind feet, make attempts to lie down, roll on its back and remain in that position for a while. The pulse increases with the pain, temperature rises from one-half to one degree, breathing labored and fast, the animal sweats in spots, there may be diarrhoea present, but this does not frequently occur.

Unfavorable symptoms of spasmodic colic are cold legs to the feet, point of the ears cold, trembling of the muscles, cold sweats, mucous membranes of the nose, mouth and eyes have a dark color due to the congestion.

TREATMENT: In all cases of spasmodic colic, except where there is diarrhoea present or mares heavily in foal, give Aloin, two drams; Ginger, two drams. Place in gelatin capsule and give with capsule gun. It is advisable to give rectal injection of Warm Water and Glycerine. They are soothing and cooling to the intestinal canal. Also give the following prescription: Pulv. Nux Vomica, four ounces; Carbonate of Ammonia, four ounces; Asafoetida, four ounces. Make into six powders; place one powder in gelatin capsule and give with capsule gun every two hours until relieved. The former prescription removes the cause as it is a physic. The latter contains medicines blended so as to counteract the spasmodic contractions of the bowels. It is also a heart stimulant, just what is needed in colic to keep up the animal's vitality. Beware of colic remedies that are given in drop doses. They contain drugs to only relieve the pain and not remove the cause. When their effects are worn off, the disease has progressed; the animal's heart action has been weakened and chances are that the animal will die. If drenching is resorted to, it must be done with great precaution. Remember a horse cannot breathe through his mouth.

SIDE BONES

CAUSE: The chief causes of Side Bones are: Deprivation of frog pressure, injuries, high heeled shoes, the use of which is almost entirely confined to draft horses. A high-heeled shoe prevents the frog from resting on the ground which is its natural support.

SYMPTOMS: Enlargement just above the hoof, usually affecting the front feet, or may affect only one side of one of the feet. The pain which produces the lameness is due to pressure on the soft tissues between the newly formed side bone and the hoof. Sometimes the enlargement has a tendency to spread the hoof. In such a case the lameness is not so severe.

TREATMENT: Clip the hair from over the Side Bone and rasp the foot below the enlargement, so that the hoof will be flexible on pressure from the fingers. Then apply the following to both the enlargement and the rasped surface on the hoof: Red Iodide of Mercury, two drams; Pulv. Cantharides, four drams. Mix well in two ounces of Lard and apply every forty-eight hours until three applications have been applied.

If you must work the animal, put it to some easy work where it has soft ground to walk upon.

STAGGERS

(Forage Poisoning--Inflammation of the Brain)

(Cerebral Meningitis)

CAUSE: Certain plants or stagnant water are most commonly instrumental in producing staggers; frequently seen in the early autumn months when the grass in the pastures becomes dry and certain forage remains green which contains toxic principles. These plants are ravenously eaten by horses on account of being green and tender. This is one of the common causes of the disease, although mouldy, indigestible or highly nitrogenous foods are frequently producers of staggers. This form of staggers is not contagious, although what produces staggers in one horse will also produce it in another. In this way several horses may become affected with staggers at the same time. Inflammation of the brain may occur as a complication of some infectious or digestive disease. Other causes are blows to the head, tumors in or on the brain, which cause the animal to naturally stagger, as the brain controls the horse's organs of locomotion.

SYMPTOMS: Vary to a certain extent, but a careful observer will detect some trouble connected with the nervous system, as the animal walking unsteadily, stepping high and keeping the legs spread apart, bracing itself to keep from falling. There is also great depression, as dullness and sleepiness with little or no inclination to move about. The head may be placed against a wall or fence and the legs kept moving as if the horse were trying to walk. As the disease progresses and no attempts are made to relieve it, they will become fractious, nervous, easily excited, pawing and eventually fall, keeping the feet moving as if walking, throwing their heads about in a delirious manner and eventually death follows. The horse as a rule eats and drinks ravenously when the first signs of staggers are noticed, but in its latter stages the tongue and gullet become paralyzed and although the animal attempts to eat and drink he cannot swallow. The pulse varies. It is strong, but subnormal when the first symptoms of staggers are noticed, that is to say, it is as slow as twenty to twenty-five beats per minute. As the disease progresses, however, it becomes weaker and faster. Constipation frequently accompanies this disease, also paleness tinged with yellow about the mucous membranes of the mouth and eyes. In many instances I believe that the poisonous forage eaten by horses depresses the heart action to such an extent that it results in the brain not receiving the proper blood supply, causing dizziness or staggers.

TREATMENT: Place the animal in a clean, dark stall, keeping the surroundings as quiet as possible. In its first stages it is easily treated, but as the horse becomes easily excited and his swallowing becomes difficult, treatment becomes more difficult. When the first signs are noticed, administer a physic as: Aloin, two or three drams; Ginger, two or three drams, according to the size of the animal. Place in gelatin capsule and give with capsule gun. This physic removes the irritant from the intestines and prevents its absorption into the blood. Also administer the following: Bromide of Potassium, twelve ounces; Nitrate of Potash, four ounces; Iodide of Potash, three ounces. Make into twenty-four capsules and give one capsule every four hours.

My method of administering medicine to animals places me in a position to treat them and compel them to take the medicine even though paralysis may exist. When animals will eat, feed food that is easily digested, as hot wheat bran mashes, steamed rolled oats and vegetables and give small quantities, but often, of clean fresh water. It is necessary to give stimulants and tonics as soon as they are on the road to recovery, as Pulv. Nux Vomica, four ounces; Pulv. Gentian Root, four ounces; Sulphate of Iron, two ounces. Make into sixteen capsules and give one capsule three times daily.

TIFLE JOINT LAMENESS

(Dislocation of the Patella)

Although dislocations are infrequent, this is the most common form which occurs in the horse.

CAUSE: Young loose jointed horses are predisposed to dislocation of the stifle on account of the comparative want of strength of their ligaments. They are much more liable to this accident than older horses, especially if they are in poor health or in rough hilly pastures; the nature of which would naturally make them susceptible to this injury, which, however, may take place as a result of accident at any age. Young horses that suffer, off and on from dislocation, often lose their liability with increasing strength and age. This dislocation may be partial or complete. In the former instance and the most common is where the patella, or the little stifle bone that glides in the groove composed of the lower hip and upper thigh bones, has become partially dislocated or removed from its natural position.

SYMPTOMS: When the dislocation is complete the affected limb is drawn forward, while the foot from the pastern down is drawn backward, and the animal may throw weight on it when made to move, which is accomplished with great difficulty. When the dislocation is partial, the symptoms are about the same as mentioned, only the limb is less rigid. If the horse is moved, the stifle makes a klick sound. In this form, you may have both limbs affected.

TREATMENT: In partial dislocation, the stifle bone may be replaced by drawing the leg forward, and with the hand pressing in on the stifle. In complete dislocation, tie a rope around the pastern of the affected leg, then draw the rope through a collar placed around the horse's neck and draw forward as far as possible and tie. Then press with both hands inward. After the stifle is placed back into position use the following liniment: Aqua Ammonia Fort., four ounces; Oil of Turpentine, four ounces; Raw Linseed Oil, four ounces. Mix and apply well over the stifle joint once or twice a day for two or three days. Feed nourishing food and put the animal to slow, easy work or turn out to good pasture.

In old chronic cases of Stifle Joint Lameness, treatment is of no value, therefore, care for the animal as soon as the catch in the walk or lameness appears.

STRING-HALT

CAUSE: Several theories have been put forth as to the cause of String-Halt which is generally supposed to be a nervous disease; a condition opposite to paralysis. The exact cause of this disease is hard to determine, but it is likely to occur in highly nervous horses. It sometimes follows an injury which may have irritated the nerves in some way. I believe that castration causes it in many instances, due to the severe struggle when being thrown, or pulling down severely on the spermatic cord when removing the testicle.

SYMPTOMS: Spasmodic contraction of one or both limbs. This sign varies, as sometimes it is very violent, while in others it may be so slight that it is hard to detect when stepping the horse forward, but on backing or turning the horse around the signs are easily noticed. All symptoms are better marked in the winter than in the summer, as some show it in the winter that do not show it in the summer at all.

TREATMENT: Very unsuccessful, although an operation proves beneficial in some cases, but if this is attempted, the services of a competent Veterinarian should be secured.

The feeding of laxative foods that are easily digested relieves String-Halt in many instances.

SORE THROAT

(Pharyngitis--Laryngitis)

CAUSE: Exposure to cold weather or rain when the animal is not accustomed to it; drenching with irritating medicines or inhaling irritating smoke or gases.

SYMPTOMS: At first the animal generally chills, the legs and ears are cold, but eventually they become very warm as the temperature increases, coughing, grinding of the teeth, saliva oozing from the mouth; the animal will hold its head in a stiff straight position, moving it as little as possible. There will be great difficulty in masticating and swallowing, as the food will come from the mouth in the form of wads, and as this soreness of the throat progresses food will also come from the nostrils. This is a bad sign, as extensive inflammation is no doubt present. Water, also, runs through the nostrils freely when the animal attempts to drink, due to the swollen condition of the throat. The animal forces the water back into the mouth, but is unable to swallow and hence the water gushes out through the nostrils. The animal evinces great pain when pressure is applied from the outside and he breathes with great difficulty. Although the pulse is not much affected at this stage, the temperature is elevated from one to two degrees above normal. The urine becomes scanty and highly colored, the eyes bloodshot and discharging. Eventually the throat becomes greatly swollen and abscesses may form and discharge. As a rule constipation is associated with this disease.

TREATMENT: Mild attacks of sore throat are easily treated, but when serious cases develop, it is unsuccessful. Place the animal in a clean, comfortable stall; permit as much fresh air as possible, but avoid all drafts. If the weather is chilly, blanket the animal, hand rub the legs and bandage with woolen cloths or bandage. Administer a mixture made from Chlorate of Potash, three ounces; Nitrate of Potash, three ounces; Tannic Acid, one-half ounce; Molasses, one-half pint; Pine Tar, one-half pint. Mix well and place about one tablespoonful on the tongue every two hours in severe cases; in mild attacks, give less frequently. When they will eat, feed food that is easily digested, as hot wheat bran mashes and steamed rolled oats containing two or three ounces of pure ground flaxseed. It is always necessary to apply strong liniments to the throat, as they relieve inflammation and stimulate the formation of an abscess. The following liniment will be found very beneficial: Aqua Ammonia Fort., four ounces; Oil of Turpentine, four ounces; Sweet Oil, six ounces; shake well and apply two or three times daily. If the swelling is extreme between the jaws, so as to interfere with the animal's breathing, it is well to lance the abscess if a soft spot can be found. Just cut through the skin with a knife; then use a clean blunt instrument to locate the pus cavity. Otherwise, severe hemorrhage may be produced.

SURFEIT

(Nettle-Rash--Urtecaria)

CAUSE: The usual cause of Surfeit is supposed to be due to a character of food consumed which upsets the animal's digestive organs, the skin being continuous with the mucous membranes lining the intestinal canal. A disturbance of the one structure is readily communicated to the other. Apparently, owing to the extreme dry nature of the forage during the greater part of the year, horses in the United States frequently suffer from Surfeit.

SYMPTOMS: Surfeit is a term applied to an eruption of small irregular lumps or boils which are more or less painful to the touch and which break out suddenly as a rule on the horse's body and neck, and in rare cases on the legs. A favorite seat of Surfeit is the parts covered with the harness or saddle and along the neck and withers. Surfeit is very troublesome and annoys both the horse and driver, especially when the horse perspires, as he will rub violently when coming in contact with any object.

TREATMENT: Give two to four ounces of Epsom Salts in hot wheat bran mashes every morning. Feed as much sloppy food as possible, vegetables, etc. Avoid feeding dry woody hay, as it irritates the intestines and aggravates the disease.

SWEENEY

(Atrophy)

CAUSE: An ill fitting collar, one tug longer than the other, striking an object when pulling, like a stone or a corner of a building, slipping, kicks, or the animal may have a splint, sprain, ringbone, side bone, coffin-joint lameness, curb, corns, stifle lameness, in fact anything that tends to make an animal favor the use of certain muscles. It is not a disease, just a lack in the development of the muscles, which waste away or shrink when not used as nature provided. For instance, perhaps you have had or have seen persons that had a fractured leg or arm and on account of not being able to use the leg or arm the muscles wasted away (Atrophy), until they were used normally for sometime, when the muscles again came back to their normal size.

SYMPTOMS: First locate the cause. The animal may be very lame although I have seen Sweeneys where lameness was very hard to detect, being those which were usually due to ill fitting collars. Remember you can have a Sweeney of the hip as well as the shoulder, and keep in mind the above mentioned causes.

TREATMENT: When you have an animal affected with Sweeney, find the true cause and remove it if possible. Unless the Sweeney is an old chronic one, it is successfully treated with Aqua Ammonia Fort., four ounces; Turpentine, four ounces; Sweet Oil, four ounces. Mix and apply well over wasted muscles once a day. If the application is too irritating, as some horses have thinner skins than others, it is advisable to add more Sweet Oil than above mentioned.

TAPEWORM

(Taenia)

These worms have been found in the horse, but so rarely that they need not be considered.

THOROUGHPIN

CAUSE: Generally due to some irritation of the hock joint such as severe sprains from animal jumping, slipping, kick or falling through a culvert or bridge or it is frequently hereditary; so be very careful in choosing a sire when breeding.

SYMPTOMS: Sometimes there is lameness when the Thoroughpin is first noticed, but it will gradually disappear as soon as the inflammation ceases. There will be a puffy, soft enlargement which occurs at the upper and back part of the hock, beneath the great tendons. Generally both sides are enlarged and puffy, but occasionally it happens that one side is only involved. Thoroughpin is also a forerunner of Bog Spavin as they generally are connected, as you are aware that the hock contains joint oil as all other joints do, retained in place by a thin, white fibrous membrane. Irritation of the hock joint tends to develop an extra large quantity of joint oil, and the hock is less protected by tendons where a Thoroughpin or Bog Spavin occurs--hence those puffy swellings are filled with joint oil and are connected. If you press on one side of a Thoroughpin, you will see the other side bulge out. If you press on a Bog Spavin and there is a Thoroughpin present, you will see it bulge on either side of the Thoroughpin--or vice versa.

TREATMENT: If on an old horse and the Thoroughpin is of long standing, treatment is unsatisfactory, but on the other hand if the animal is young it can be successfully treated with Tincture of Iodine, one ounce; Gum Camphor, two ounces; Gasolene, one pint. Mix well and rub in with nail or tooth brush twice a week. Keep the animal as quiet as possible as the results will be accomplished much sooner. Never attempt to open or lance a puffy swelling about a joint as it contains joint oil. The result would be an open joint.

THRUSH

CAUSE: The two main causes of Thrush are lack of pressure on the frog and the decomposing effect of filth and fermentation of organic matter which accumulates in the cleft of the frog.

SYMPTOMS: The animal in some cases is lame; there will be a swelling accompanied by a very fetid discharge; in some cases the frog has practically rotted away; there will be more or less inflammation in the foot. The legs may even swell. Thrush is more frequently found in the hind feet because of the manure and filth with which they must come in contact.

TREATMENT: Cut away all loose pieces of horn from over the frog and apply a Flaxseed meal poultice and leave it on for twenty-four hours, after which wash well with Soap and warm water. Then apply Calomel to the groove in the frog. Keep the foot clean. Do not allow the animal to stand in filth.

WIND COLIC

(Flatulent Colic)

CAUSE: This dangerous form of Colic is a distension of the bowels with gas, resulting generally from the decomposition of undigested food in the bowels. It sometimes follows Spasmodic Colic, in which there is first spasms due to the irritations set up by the presence of undigested matter, and subsequently this food decomposes and forms gas. I may conclude that Flatulent or Wind Colic is usually caused by errors in feeding and watering horses. Perhaps the animal has been given large quantities of rank grass, watery roots, which on account of its moist nature is quickly swallowed without being properly masticated.

SYMPTOMS: The signs resemble those of Spasmodic Colic, except that they are less violent. In most cases there is general accumulation of gas, the abdomen distended to a considerable size before the animal shows signs of uneasiness. In cases where the animal swells on the right side, it is the large intestines filled with gas. In other cases where both sides are equally swollen, the stomach and small intestines contain gas. The horse's back will have an arched appearance, passing of gas from the anus frequently, the horse will make attempts to vomit. In some cases actual vomiting takes place. This is a bad sign, as rupture of the stomach usually occurs at this stage.

TREATMENT: Give Aloin, two drams; Ginger, two drams, in gelatin capsule and give with capsule gun. However, this is a physic and should not be given to mares heavily in foal. Also apply to the abdominal cavity, liniment consisting of Aqua Ammonia Fort., four ounces; Oil of Turpentine, four ounces; Sweet Oil, four ounces. Mix and rub in well over the abdomen.

To mares heavy with foal, apply the above liniment and give rectal injections of Glycerine and warm water frequently.

The following remedy should be administered to all cases of Colic, including mares heavy with foal: Aromatic Spirits of Ammonia, six ounces; Turpentine, six ounces. Mix well together and place one ounce in gelatin capsule and give with capsule gun every hour. Puncturing the intestines is advisable in some cases to relieve them of gas. This requires a special instrument for the purpose and no one should attempt to perform the operation unless they know the anatomy of the part, as the arteries of the intestines may be penetrated and produce internal hemorrhage or infection of the intestines, or abscesses may follow.

WIND GALLS

CAUSE: By concussions from fast work on hard roads and from sprains from slipping.

SYMPTOMS: When concussions alone are responsible, the suspensory ligament and the back tendons will at first be in a normal condition, and the swelling will probably be confined to both the inside and outside of the leg, and may be felt in the form of a puffy swelling on each side of the fetlock by placing the fore finger and the thumb on the joint. In more serious cases resulting from sprains, the vacant space between the back tendons and the suspensory ligament may also become filled with fluids. In other words, a Wind Gall has formed. In some cases the animal may be lame.

TREATMENT: When there is heat present apply cold, wet packs until the heat disappears. Then apply Tincture of Iodine, one ounce; Gum Camphor, two ounces; to one pint of Gasolene. Apply every three days with nail or tooth brush. Shake contents of the bottle well each time before applying.

I may add that this is a very difficult blemish to treat and is not always successful, so do not be discouraged if the enlargements do not disappear, but the above prescription has proven the most successful of any treatment I have personally used in my private practice.

WOLF OR SUPERNUMERARY TEETH

Wolf Teeth are comparatively small in size and have only one root and are found just in front of the upper molar teeth. Sometimes they do harm, but that is an exception and not the rule. They can be easily removed with a pair of small forceps or they may be punched out in some instances.

I think they interfere with the eyes, causing them to become watery and inflamed due to the tooth exerting some influence upon the ophthalmic division of the fifth nerve.

Supernumerary Teeth: Tooth substance may develop in almost any part of the body. These are called Supernumerary Teeth and are most commonly found in the testicles, ovaries and sinuses of the head, etc.

WOUNDS

Wounds caused by external injuries have a general resemblance, and whether clean-cut, punctured, lacerated, poisonous, gunshot, etc., require practically the same treatment.

TREATMENT: Wash with a Carbolic solution, one tablespoonful to one pint of distilled water.

SEWING OF WOUNDS: I cannot say that I am in favor of sewing wounds unless they are gaping or wide open.

After the wound is washed, dust with Iodoform, Boracic Acid and Tannic Acid, each one ounce. Powder finely and place in a sifter top can and apply twice daily. Cord or heavy thread may be used for sewing the wound after being saturated in a Carbolic Acid solution, using a large darning needle. If the animal is vicious, place a twitch on his nose or it may be necessary to throw him.

DISEASES OF CATTLE

Causes, Symptoms and Treatments

1. Mouth 2. Nostrils 3. Muzzle 4. Face 5. Eyes 6. Forehead 7. Ears 6. Poll 9. Horns 10. Jaws 11. Dewlap 12. Brisket 13. Neck 14. Withers 15. Crops 16. Shoulders 17. Heart Girth 18. Fore flank 19. Legs 20. Feet 21. Dew claws 22. Belly 23. Milk wells 24. Milk veins 25. Fore udder 26. Teats 27. Barrel or ribs 28. Back 29. Coupling 30. Rear Flanks 31. Hook points 32. Tail-head 33. Pin

bones or thurls 34. Rump 35. Esoutcheon 36. Tail 37. Thighs 38. Rear Udder 39. Switch

CHAPTER II

ABSCESSES

CAUSE: Bruises and injuries. They are also seen in complication with various other diseases, as Laryngitis, Pharyngitis, Tuberculosis, Lump Jaw, Blood Poison or Pyemia and Septicemia.

SYMPTOMS: Symptoms will vary according to the nature of the disease or injury. It may not be noticed at first, but upon careful examination swollen lines will be observed running from the point of swelling. In many cases a swelling is noticed which is hot, painful and throbbing, which enlarges rapidly in two or three days. The swelling and heat gradually disappear but the Abscess continues to grow. The hair falls from the point of swelling and in a short time breaks and discharges pus. The cavity gradually fills up and heals by granulation.

TREATMENT: In all cases, hasten the ripening process as much as possible by applying hot water packs or hot bran, flaxseed or vegetable poultices. It is common with Veterinarians to lance an Abscess as soon as possible, but this requires considerable skill and practice and I would advise stock owners to be very cautious when performing this operation, as there is great danger of cutting arteries which would cause excessive bleeding. A very good plan is to encourage the full ripening of an Abscess, as above stated. When opened, do not squeeze the Abscess to any extent, but press gently with clean hands or cloth to remove the core or clot. After this, just simply keep the Abscess open by washing with a three per cent Carbolic Acid solution, or Bichloride of Mercury, one in one thousand solution. Hyposulphite of Soda in ounce doses should be given two or three times a day in their drinking water. This will prevent the absorption of impurities from the abscess into the blood circulation.

ABORTION

(Non-Contagious)

CAUSE: Injuries from slipping or falling on icy roads, in box cars, and deep gutters; receiving blows on the body, keeping the animal in insanitary stables, eating poor food that may be irritating or poisonous, etc. In such cases, the cow's vitality is low so that the foetus dies and is expelled as a result. Losing large quantities of blood also produces Abortion, or a cow heavy with calf, on being placed in the same quarters with the cows that retain their afterbirth, is liable to abort. Intestinal worms, lung worms, liver flukes, causing an excessive drain upon the system or producing irritation of the digestive organs, in consequence of which cow gets very poor and emaciated. The above mentioned are perhaps the most common causes of "Non-Contagious Abortion."

SYMPTOMS: The cow is uneasy, becomes separated from the herd, the bag and vagina may be slightly inflamed and perhaps the latter discharging. If a cow heavy with calf craves the chewing and eating of dirt, rags, nails, etc., this is a sign of a lack of iron or phosphorus in her system and food containing these elements should be provided.

PREVENTIVE TREATMENT: Provide clean, warm, comfortable quarters, good food, pure water to drink, do not subject her to any injuries, do not permit her coming in contact with cows retaining their afterbirth.

The above mentioned is very important, especially if the cows are valuable and a large yield of milk is expected. If they have worms, treat the same as under their special heading. If they have a loss of blood or a lack of mineral matter in their system, the following is very efficient: Pulv. Ferri Sulphate, four ounces; Pulv. Nux Vomica, two ounces; Pulv. Fenugreek Seed, four ounces. Mix and make into sixteen powders. Give one powder two or three times a day in feed or place in a gelatin capsule and give with capsule gun.

AMAUROSIS OF THE EYE

CAUSE: Paralysis of the optic nerve.

SYMPTOMS: Pupil fully dilated and of a glassy appearance. This condition is sometimes called "Glass Eye." The cow carries the head high and steps high. This condition is very uncommon in cattle.

TREATMENT: Nothing can be done for a cow if she is blind, but this condition may be prevented if detected in its early stages of development by the proper feeding of nourishing food, good clean surroundings and the administration of nerve tonics, as Pulv. Nux Vomica, four ounces; Pulv. Gentian Root, four ounces; Potassium Iodide, three ounces. Make into twenty-four powders and place one powder in feed two or three times daily; or make into twenty-four capsules and give one capsule two or three times a day with capsule gun.

ANTHRAX

Anthrax is a very contagious disease and is communicable to all warm blooded animals and man.

CAUSE: Due to the presence of a germ called the Bacillus of Anthrax and is one of the oldest diseases attributed to germs. These Bacilli thrive in warm climates, although found in cold countries. The infection is carried to various parts of the world by box-cars, ships, hides, hoofs, horns, wool and hair taken from sick or dead animals affected with Anthrax. This, perhaps, is the most common method of spreading the disease.

SYMPTOMS: Loss of appetite, grinding of the teeth indicating great pain, trembling of the muscles, temperature elevated to 104 or 106 degrees F., breathing very rapid, pulse fast and weak, hair rough. There are some cases where the animals are seized quickly with the disease and die very suddenly. This form resembles apoplexy. Carbuncles or Abscesses are seen on the surface of the body in nearly all cases, also a bloody discharge from the mouth and nose. The animal may stamp the ground, rear in the air, run and finally go into convulsions and die. This is termed "the furious form of Anthrax."

TREATMENT: Prevention is the most important. Fields or pastures that are infected with this disease should be burned every summer if possible, to destroy the germs. The animals that succumb to the disease should be buried deeply and quicklime thrown upon them, also any blood stains upon the ground should have a strong disinfectant thrown upon them. The hide of such an animal should not be used as the person removing it is likely to contract the same disease, especially if an abrasion is present on the hand, or such a hide or any portion thereof is likely to spread the infection after reaching the tannery, etc.

MEDICAL TREATMENT OR SERUM TREATMENT: This is the only thorough method of eradicating the disease, and when this disease once becomes prevalent in a locality the services of a competent Veterinarian should be secured and all the animals inoculated.

BARRENNESS

(Failure to Breed)

CAUSE: Wasting or Atrophy, chronic inflammation of the mucous membrane lining the organs of generation, Whites, absence or excessive secretions of the organs of generation, contraction or displacement of the womb, horns being telescoped or twisted, cysts or growths of the ovaries, in-breeding or being a twin, are the predisposing causes of Barrenness.

TREATMENT: Unsuccessful as a rule. Unless the cow is very valuable, treatment is not advisable. A careful examination, however, is recommended. If due to contraction of the neck of the womb it can be readily dilated by the use of the hand, after being greased with Carbolated Sweet Oil before attempting to perform the operation.

BLACK LEG

(Symptomatic Anthrax--Black Quarter)

CAUSE: Due to germs. The Bacillus of Black Leg perhaps gains entrance to the blood by wounds of the skin or the mucous membranes lining the mouth and the intestines. This disease principally affects cattle, although sheep and goats may become affected with the same disease.

SYMPTOMS: This disease affects cattle that are in good condition between the ages of six months and two years. In most cases death is very sudden, and perhaps the animal is found dead. The first symptoms are high temperatures from 104 to 108 degrees F., loss of appetite, the animal stops chewing the cud, breathing considerably hurried, the joints of the limbs become swollen, also the chest and shoulders. All the swellings are painful on pressure and spread very rapidly over the body. The affected animals move with great difficulty and lie down frequently. If the hand is passed over the body, there is a peculiar crackling sound due to the gas developing under the skin. At the most distended portions of the swellings, the skin becomes dry and the animal apparently has no sense of feeling. If the skin is punctured at this place, there will be a dark-red, frothy discharge which has a very disagreeable odor. There will be a shivering of the muscles and the animal dies from convulsions.

TREATMENT: Remove non-affected animals to non-infected pastures, and confine affected animals to as small a territory as possible. The carcasses of the dead animals should be buried deep and covered with lime or burned, being very careful that all blood stains on the ground where the animals have been skinned are thoroughly disinfected. Inoculation is necessary, and is the best form of treatment in localities where Black Leg exists. Inoculate or vaccinate the calves when six months old or over, although after the animal reaches the age of two years or over they generally become immune from this disease.

BLEEDING

(Hemorrhage)

CAUSE: Sometimes bleeding follows dehorning, castration, and wounds due to various other causes.

TREATMENT: When bleeding from a large artery, it should be tied with a clean silk or linen thread or twisted with a pair of forceps or cauterized with a hot iron. Sometimes compression by the use of tightly bound bandages proves effective, although the former appliances are more practical. Tincture Chloride of Iron applied to small arteries or veins causes the blood to clot in the arteries or veins and hence stops the Hemorrhage. It is very essential that all wounds should be treated antiseptically and I cannot say that I favor washing a wound with water only in cases where the wound is very filthy, and I prefer powder applications in preference to any other antiseptics. The following will be found very effective in the treatment of the majority of wounds: Boracic Acid, two ounces; Iodoform, two drams; Tannic Acid, one-half ounce; Calomel, one dram. Powder finely and mix well. Place in sifter top can and apply two or three times daily.

BLOATING

A very common disorder in cattle and characterized by a puffed up appearance of the left flank. The cow has four stomachs of which the rumen is the largest, its capacity being about fifty gallons in the average cow, and it is this stomach which fills with gas when a cow bloats.

CAUSE: Eating green clover or alfalfa; even when a cow is accustomed to this diet, it may cause bloating if wet with dew or rain; cured alfalfa, moldy or frozen mangles will also produce bloating; the above mentioned foods undergo a process of fermentation which causes excessive formation of gas, and death may result very quickly and may be due to rupture of the stomach or the diaphragm (muscle separating the abdominal and lung cavities), but is more often due to suffocation caused by the distension of the stomach which becomes so large that it presses the diaphragm forward against the lungs in such a manner as to stop their movement and the animal smothers. When the cow falls, it indicates that one of these possibilities has occurred and death follows quickly.

SYMPTOMS: Cattle usually bloat suddenly and without warning; the left flank becomes abnormally swollen; back is arched, breathing labored; sometimes the tongue hangs out and the animal bellows. When rupture or suffocation occurs the animal reels, staggers, and falls, after which nothing more can be done.

TREATMENT: No time should be lost. Where the stomach is enormously distended with gas so as to cause the animals to stagger and breathe very rapidly, they should be gagged. This can be easily accomplished by taking a piece of wood about two inches in diameter, and eight inches to one foot long, placing it in their mouth and retaining it in that position by tying a string on each end and placing it back of the ears. If this does not give relief immediately, puncture the left flank about five inches downward and forward from the angle of hip bone. However, puncturing should not be resorted to only in cases where death threatens the animal, as abscesses, infection and severe hemorrhage may follow. A very reliable medical treatment for this condition should be in the medicine chest of every stockman, such as Pulv. Asafetida, Oil of Turpentine, each one ounce. Place in gelatin capsules. This is a very efficient remedy for the eradication of excessive fermentation of gases in the stomach or bloating.

BLOOD POISON

(Pyemia-Septicaemia)

CAUSE: Due to a septic infection taken into the blood, frequently found in cows with retained afterbirths, following inflammation of the womb or intestines, wounds and bruises of the skin and frequently found in calves affected with Joint Ill.

SYMPTOMS: High temperature 103 to 107 degrees F., pulse rapid and feeble, breathing increased, grinding of the teeth, the animal refuses to eat in most cases and ceases to chew the cud, although there may be great thirst present. Abscesses may form in various parts of the body, the membranes of the eyes and mouth will be injected with blood, giving them a dark-red appearance, although in the latter stages of Blood Poison this may change to a yellowish tinge. Constipation or Diarrhoea may be connected with the disease. The animal dies by general emaciation from four to six days after the first symptoms are noticed.

TREATMENT: Unsuccessful, as when the infection once becomes absorbed in the blood it is always certain that death will follow. If due to injuries or wounds, wash them with Bichloride solution, one part to one thousand parts of water, but if due to retained afterbirth or inflammation of the womb, inject one gallon of distilled water containing five per cent Carbolic Acid. If in young calves, treat the same as under the heading of Joint Ill. If due to inflammation of the intestines, give Hyposulphite of Soda, two ounces; Potassi Iodide, one dram, two or three times a day in their drinking water. When abscesses form, lance them with a clean, sharp knife. If the animal is constipated place two drams of Aloin, two drams of Pulv. Gentian Root in a capsule and give with capsule gun. If Diarrhoea is present give Gum Catechu, two drams; Protan, three drams; Zinc Sulphocarbolates, one grain. Place in gelatin capsule and give with capsule gun. Feed warm wheat bran mashes, steamed rolled oats, vegetables and green grass, if possible.

BLOODY FLUX

(Dysentery)

CAUSE: Chilling of the outer surface of the body. Improper feeding, as contaminated food or water, sometimes connected with parasitic diseases of the intestines.

SYMPTOMS: Dysentery is a sign of some irritation of the intestines terminating into increased contractions of muscular fibers of the bowels. The fecal matter, if frequently expelled, at first consists of a thick feces, but as the disease progresses the fecal matter becomes very thin and watery and tinged with blood and very offensive. When the first signs are noticed the animals show no constitutional disturbances, but later they exhibit abdominal pain by looking around to the flank. At this stage they are very weak, throwing the feet well together, giving the back an arched appearance, and are very uneasy although they may lie down frequently. Temperature elevated from one to three degrees. The animal becomes emaciated and eventually dies.

TREATMENT: Determine the cause and remove it if possible. Keep the animal quiet. Give pure water to drink in small quantities but often. If the animal will eat, feed steamed rolled oats, etc. Flaxseed tea is very beneficial, as it is soothing to the intestines and assists in removing the irritations. Pour one quart of boiling water on one-half pint of pure Flaxseed, allowing it to cool, then compel the animal to drink it. The following prescription will be found very effective in all forms of Diarrhoea: Tannic Acid, one ounce; Protan, two ounces; Gum Catechu, two ounces; Beechwood Creosote, four scruples; Zinc Sulphocarbolates, eight grains. Make into eight capsules and give one capsule every three or four hours with capsule gun.

BLOODY MILK

CAUSE: Bloody Milk may be the result of injury, congestion, inflammation of the udder. Feeding on rich milk-producing food suddenly may produce it. Bloody Milk is also produced in a cow by excitement when in heat or from eating resinous plants or shrubs.

TREATMENT: It is advisable in most cases to give a physic consisting of two drams of Aloin and Ginger two drams. Also administer Potassium Nitrate, four ounces; Potassium Chlorate, two ounces, made into eight capsules and give one capsule twice daily with capsule gun. If due to rich food, reduce it. If due to eating resinous plants, remove them from the pasture containing such shrubbery. Where congestion or inflammation of the bag is thought to produce it, apply Hot Water Packs, then dry and apply Blue Ointment and Camphorated Ointment, equal parts, two ounces. Mix well and rub on thoroughly two or three times a day.

BLUE MILK

CAUSE: This condition is due to a germ (the Bacillus Cyanogenes) which may occur in rich milk or cream immediately after being drawn or the germ may find its way into the opening of the teat.

TREATMENT: Injections into the teat of a solution composed of the following: Hyposulphite of Soda, two drams; Boracic Acid, one dram, dissolved in one pint of boiling water. Permit to cool and inject a small quantity in each teat once or twice a day for three or four days. This will destroy the Blue Milk producing germ without any injuries to the cow, udder or teats.

BRONCHITIS

CAUSE: Inhaling irritating gases or foreign bodies. It is commonly seen after drenching from liquid escaping into the windpipe instead of going down the gullet. Animals exposed to cold, wet weather when not accustomed to it frequently develop Bronchitis.

SYMPTOMS: Loss of appetite, chilling, temperature elevated two or three degrees above normal; ears and legs cold, nose hot and dry, breathing short and labored, painful coughing, slight discharge from the nostrils and saliva oozing from the mouth. If the ear is placed over the lower portion of the neck, a crepitating sound can be heard.

TREATMENT: Place the animal in a clean, comfortable stall where there is pure air and light but no drafts. Clothe the body if the weather is cold. Hand rub the legs and bandage with woolen cloths. Give inhalations of steam from Hot Water and Pine Tar for twenty minutes two or three times a day. Also administer Nux Vomica, four ounces; Ginger, four ounces; Nitrate of Potash, four ounces. Make into sixteen capsules and give one capsule every four hours. Applications of the following liniment are of some value: Aqua Ammonia Fort., three ounces; Oil of Turpentine, three ounces; Sweet Oil, six ounces. Apply over the region of the windpipe the full length of the neck.

CALF SCOURS

(Cholera--White Scours--Bloody Flux)

CAUSE: It is produced by a specific germ and is communicated by direct or indirect contact with the germ which may gain entrance into the blood by the umbilical cord at or shortly after birth or through the digestive canal by drinking milk or eating food contaminated with the disease-producing germ. The more common means of spreading the disease is through pails, drinking troughs, etc.

SYMPTOMS: One of the most deadly forms of Diarrhoea. This usually appears a few days after birth, although in some cases it takes several days for it to develop. Every sign of Diarrhoea is present, as frequent passages of feces of a yellowish-white color, frothy and very offensive in odor. The calf is very dull, weak, back arched, hair rough, eyes glassy and sunken back in their sockets, belly retracted, breathing short and fast. The calf finally lies flat on the side, head resting on the floor or ground with a temperature generally below normal. The calf finally becomes unconscious and death follows.

TREATMENT: Give Protan, three ounces; Zinc Sulphocarbolates, eight grains; Gum Catechu, powdered, two ounces; Ginger, one ounce; Beechwood Creosote, one dram. Make into eight capsules and give one capsule every two hours until relieved. When the calf will take its feed, if not nursing its mother, see that the milk is pure and the utensil containing it thoroughly scalded with hot water. Keep the animal in clean, sanitary quarters, as quiet as possible for a few days, and if the disease is not too far advanced a good recovery will follow.

CALVING

Signs of Normal Calving are firmness and enlargement of the udder, extending well forward following the milk veins. The teats as a rule discharge a thin milky fluid, relaxation of the muscles on each side of the croup or the base of the tail. The outer surface of the womb becomes swollen and inflamed, discharging sticky, stringy, transparent mucus. The cow becomes uneasy, stops eating, and if in a pasture becomes separated from the rest of the herd; will lie down and get up alternately as if in great agony. When birth pains start, the back is arched, and a severe straining follows the contraction of the abdominal muscles. The membranes covering the foetus will be the first to make their appearance, engorged with a fluid from the womb. This is commonly known as the water bag, which eventually bursts and the two fore feet can be seen, and, as the animal continues to strain, the nose and head will be next to be seen. When the calf's shoulders are exposed, the cow as a rule rises suddenly to her feet and the entire calf is expelled, also the membranes surrounding it, but the membranes next to the womb, as a general rule, remain longer and sometimes require artificial assistance to remove them. (See Retention of the Afterbirth.) Destroy the foetal membranes by burning or burying them deeply. Do not permit the cow to eat them. Wash the calf's navel with Bichloride of Mercury, one part to one thousand parts water, once or twice a day until the navel is thoroughly dry, as an infection may follow, producing Joint Ill or Scours, from which death may result.

ABNORMAL CALVING: This is a condition where the foetus is not normally presented, as that just described. Their feet may be presented in a normal manner, but the head and neck twisted back or to one side, or the head and one fore foot may be presented normally, while the other fore foot is doubled back, or there may be a breech presentation as the rump of a foetus with both hind feet thrown close to its body. This is a very difficult presentation, especially if in a young animal. A foetus abnormally presented requires good judgment and cleanliness, also lubrication of the walls of the womb with unsalted Lard, Cotton or Sweet Oil. Endeavor to place the foetus in as near a normal position as possible before any force is used in its delivery, although where both hind feet are presented, it is advisable to remove it in this position. The hands and ropes should be clean and washed with a five per cent solution of Carbolic Acid. It is not only dangerous to the animal, but to the operator as well, if proper antiseptic precautions are not practiced.

Space does not permit me going into details on various foetal presentations nor does it permit me to explain the exact methods or operations I would use in each particular case. Nevertheless, good judgment and cleanliness are important. Do not hurry. Take your time, and you will be successful in most cases.

When the foetus is removed, and the afterbirth does not come away within twelve or eighteen hours, remove it. (See Retention of Afterbirth, which will describe its means of attachment and its removal.)

CASTING THE WITHERS

(Eversion of the Womb)

CAUSE: Failure of the womb to contract after Calving. If the womb contracts naturally and the afterbirth expelled, the cavity of the womb is nearly closed and the neck of the womb becomes so narrow that the hand cannot be inserted. When the womb fails to contract, one or both horns of the womb become so relaxed that they fall into the cavity causing straining and contraction of the abdominal muscles, forcing the womb out gradually until the organ is turned inside out. The womb can be easily distinguished from the other membranes on account of the presence of sixty to eighty mushroom-like bodies (cotyledons) two to four inches in diameter attached to the walls of the womb by a narrow neck. The womb when hanging out becomes engorged with blood and inflamed until it is as large as a grain sack, very dark in color, tears and bleeds with the slightest touch. Later it becomes lacerated and gangrenous.

SYMPTOMS: At first, the general health is not very much interfered with, but the inflammation which is marked by an elevation in temperature becomes very noticeable, accompanied by severe straining and exhaustion. The animal lies down, but continues to strain until death, unless relief is afforded the animal at once.

TREATMENT: Great care must be exercised. The parts of the womb coming in contact with the cow's hips, tail or floors must be thoroughly washed with a five per cent solution of Carbolic Acid, using a soft cloth or sponge to remove dirt, clots, etc. Place the cow in a position so as to have her hind quarters much higher than the head, and then endeavor to replace the womb. After washing as stated above, bandage the tail with a clean cloth; have an assistant hold up the womb and the operator use gentle manipulation and pressure with clean hands; this perhaps is the best method of replacing the womb. Then follow by flushing out the womb with a weak Carbolic Acid solution and luke warm water. This has a tendency to straighten out the horns of the uterus and prevent infection. If the cow continues to strain, give Potassium Bromide in ounce doses every two or three hours in her drinking water, or place in capsule and give with capsule gun.

Sometimes stimulants and tonics are necessary and the following will be found very effective: Pulv. Nux Vomica, four ounces; Pulv. Gentian Root, four ounces; Pulv. Ferri Sulphate, four ounces. Make into sixteen capsules and give one capsule every six hours with capsule gun.

It is well to compel the animal to stand or lie with the hind parts elevated, until the signs of straining have ceased.

CATARACT OF THE EYE

CAUSE: Is due to deep seated inflammation of the eye produced by an injury or weakened condition of the optic nerve.

SYMPTOMS: If the pupil of one of the eyes appears larger than the other it is well to make a careful examination, as this is the first sign of Cataract. If such a condition is neglected, partial or complete blindness will follow and a white, pearly deposit can be seen on the lens of the eye.

TREATMENT: Very unsatisfactory unless treated carefully when the first signs are noticed. Place the animal in a darkened stable. Feed clean, sloppy food and it may be necessary to give a physic consisting of two drams of Aloin, two drams of Pulv. Ginger, placed in a capsule and given with capsule gun. The following ointment, Yellow Oxide of Mercury, four grains; Lanolin, one ounce, should be mixed well and applied to the eye two or three times a day.

CATARRH

CAUSE: Ill ventilated stables, inhalations of irritating gases or sudden exposure to cold, wet weather, after being accustomed to warm stables. Most commonly seen in the Spring or Fall.

SYMPTOMS: Chilling and temperature elevated one or two degrees, pulse not much affected, breathing hurried to some extent, sneezing, coughing, dullness and the appetite is slightly impaired. In the first stages the nostrils are very dry and considerably inflamed, but in the course of a few days the fever subsides and a profuse discharge from the nose is observed.

TREATMENT: Place the animal in dry, well ventilated stall, blanket well and supply a good quality and quantity of bedding. Give inhalations from steam and hot water and Pine Tar. If the animal is constipated, give rectal injections of Soap and Warm Water two or three times a day. Also administer Potassium Nitrate, Pulv. Nux Vomica, each four ounces; Capsicum, two ounces, and Pulv. Ginger two ounces. Make into twenty-four capsules and give one capsule three or four times a day. This should not be neglected, as neglected Catarrh is liable to be followed by Laryngitis, Bronchitis, Pneumonia, Pleurisy or other diseases of the organs of breathing, which are very serious and sometimes cause the death of the animal.

CHAPPED TEATS

CAUSE: Anything that tends to irritate them. A sudden chilling of the teat in cold weather after the calf has just let it go, or after the operation of milking with wet hands or from an animal wading through deep water or tall wet grass. Also filth or irritants coming in contact with teats when lying down.

TREATMENT: Remove the cause if possible and dry the teats well after each milking and apply Zinc Oxide ointment. Feed laxative food that is easily digested, as it has a very good effect on the blood, consequently it promotes the healing of wounds.

CHOKING

(Obstruction of the Esophagus)

CAUSE: An obstruction of the Esophagus (gullet) produced by an animal attempting to swallow apples, potatoes, roots, dry grain, etc.

SYMPTOMS: A stringy discharge of saliva from the mouth, violent coughing, wrenching of the head and neck. The animal will bloat very quickly if the Esophagus or gullet is completely obstructed.

TREATMENT: The obstruction as a rule is easily located, and as quickly as possible withdraw the obstruction by inserting the hand and extracting the object. Do not attempt to push the object down into the stomach, except as a last resort, as there is a great deal of danger of rupturing the Esophagus or gullet. Push the object upward by gentle manipulation from the outside. If this fails, a smooth piece of hose about eight or nine feet long, well greased with Lard, Butter or Oil, should be passed down the Esophagus or gullet. A block of wood about two inches in diameter with a hole bored through the center just a little larger than the hose, placed in the mouth, will prevent the animal from biting the hose, and make the operation easier.

When the animal is bloated severely, puncture with a knife about four or five inches from the point of the hip downward and forward.

CHRONIC DYSENTERY

(Bacterial Dysentery--Jones Disease)

CAUSE: Acid-fast Bacillus resembling the Tubercular Bacillus that invade the intestines by the way of the animal drinking water or eating food containing the Acid-fast Bacteria.

SYMPTOMS: Diarrhoea, loss of flesh, although the appetite is good, hair becomes dry and harsh, temperature remains about normal. The Diarrhoea becomes persistent and tinged with blood. The animal becomes emaciated and anemic, exhausted, and death follows. This disease may continue for a month or even a year before death takes place. However this is very uncommon. They generally die very shortly.

TREATMENT: Separate the affected cattle from the healthy ones. All fecal matter should be deeply buried or burned, the stalls, barnyards, also thoroughly disinfected. Administration of medicine thus far has been unsatisfactory, although a treatment should be directed toward the intestines with internal antiseptics such as Zinc Sulphocarbolates, one and one-half grains; Protan, three drams; Pulv. Nux Vomica, one dram; Bismuth Subnitrate, one dram. Place in gelatin capsule and give with capsule gun. This dose should be repeated three or four times a day. Feed a good quality of food, such as wheat bran mashes or steamed rolled oats and see that the water supply is fresh and non-contaminated.

COLIC

CAUSE: Drinking large quantities of cold water when overheated. However, this disorder is very uncommon in cattle owing to the fact that they are not worked, seldom overheated and drink water very slowly.

SYMPTOMS: Kicking or raising of the feet to the belly. Lying down and getting up alternately. Distention of the stomach or paunch with gas. The animal chills or shivers, etc.

TREATMENT: Strong stimulants or tonics as the following will give immediate results if administered in its first stages: Pulv. Nux Vomica, two ounces; Pulv. Ginger, two ounces; Pulv. Capsicum, two ounces. Make into eight capsules and give one capsule every two hours until relieved. Give the capsules with capsule gun. If severe bloating accompanies a case of Colic in cattle place one ounce dose of Oil of Turpentine in ounce capsules and give with capsule gun.

CONGESTION OF THE LUNGS

CAUSE: Cattle permitted to stand in drafts when warm after being driven, etc., irritating drugs escaping into the lungs when drenching, as it is very difficult for cattle to swallow when their heads are elevated.

SYMPTOMS: Dullness. The animal loses its spirits, so to speak, usually shivers or trembles. When this ceases, the temperature rises to perhaps 105 or 106 degrees F. The ears and legs grow cold, the nose hot and dry, pulse rapid but firm, breathing short and labored, a short hacking cough will be present. Such animals generally remain standing.

Other symptoms are constipation, the feces covered with mucus or a slime, great thirst. The eyes are inflamed and look glassy. The secretions of milk are suppressed, if these symptoms develop in milking cows.

TREATMENT: Place the animal in clean, warm, comfortable quarters permitting light and as much pure air as possible, but avoid drafts and blanket the animal if chilly. Hand rub the legs and bandage with woolen cloths. Administer Pulv. Carbonate of Ammonia, four ounces; Pulv. Nux Vomica, three ounces; Quinine, two ounces; Nitrate of Potash, two ounces; Potassium Iodide, one ounce. Make into twenty-four capsules and give one capsule every four hours with capsule gun. Also apply a paste made from Mustard and cold water over the lung cavities just back of the fore legs. Apply once a day and perhaps one or two applications will be sufficient.

If this disease is treated when the first symptoms develop, a good recovery will follow. Feed easily digested food as hot wheat bran mashes or steamed rolled oats, vegetables and green grass if possible.

CONTAGIOUS ABORTION

(Infectious Abortion)

CAUSE: Due to a germ (Bacillus Abortus) coming in direct contact with the genital organs of a bull or cow and can be indefinitely transmitted from one herd to another by infected bulls serving healthy cows, or infected cows when served transmit the infection to healthy bulls. Healthy cows become infected by their genital organs coming in contact with litter on floors when lying down or rubbing against fences, walls or posts previously soiled by aborting cows. Cattle licking one another is also a prolific cause.

SYMPTOMS: The signs of calving are not so well marked as in normal calving, especially where the aborting animal is a heifer and the gestation period has not exceeded three or four weeks. In cows, especially where the gestation period has advanced to five or seven months, the symptoms are easily detected as a rule by a swelling of the udder, or what is commonly termed "making bag," the outer portions of the womb swollen and inflamed as in normal calving. As the period of abortion approaches, there will be a discharge of mucus and blood from the womb. Labor pains are not as severe as in normal calving, owing to the absence of hair on the foetus and being smaller; although the afterbirth (foetal membranes), may be retained the same as in normal calving.

PREVENTIVE TREATMENT: This perhaps is the cheapest and best method of treating Contagious Abortion. When purchasing bulls or cows, ascertain whether the farm you purchased from has Contagious Abortion. An investigation of this kind often saves labor, time and money.

MEDICAL TREATMENT: When once Contagious Abortion makes its appearance, separate infected from non-infected animals, remove all litter, manure, etc., from barns, corrals, and burn or bury deeply. The conveyances used should be tight so as to prevent scattering. Scrub and disinfect floors, fences, walls of barns and rubbing posts with a solution made from three pounds of Copper Sulphate to ten gallons of water, permitting it to thoroughly dissolve before using. Use an ordinary barrel and cover so as to prevent any cattle drinking same, as it is very poisonous. When a cow aborts, remove the calf and afterbirth in a tight receptacle that will prevent any portion from being scattered, and burn or bury deeply; disinfect the floor and walls of stall where the abortion took place as long as the cow is discharging any fluids from the womb. A gallon of distilled or boiled water containing about one per cent Carbolic Acid should be injected into the womb with an ordinary hose and funnel. This should be repeated once a day for a week. Use a solution of the same strength for washing the tail and parts around the outer part of the womb, or in fact any part that the discharge of an aborting cow may come in contact with.

Internally, give Methylen Blue in thirty grain doses, every other day for two weeks. This is an exceptionally disagreeable drug to administer as it stains everything it comes in contact with. Place it in a gelatin capsule or have your druggist prepare six or seven capsules containing thirty grains each. Then administer with capsule gun. Insist on pure Methylen Blue, accept no substitute. This treatment has proven very effective in many localities where strict aseptic precautions were carried out, as washing out the womb or any parts that the discharge of an aborting cow may come in contact with and proper cleanliness and disinfection of stables, etc. Cows should not be bred for several weeks following abortion or as long as there is a discharge present. Bulls should be treated in much the same way, as administering Methylen

Blue in same size doses for the same length of time as that of the cow. But in addition to this, use a one per cent solution of Carbolic Acid for injecting into the bull's sheath, holding the end of the sheath while the solution is being injected, until it is well distended; holding the opening of the sheath allowing the solution to remain as long as convenient. Also, wash belly, muzzle, etc., with a solution of the same strength.

COUGH

(Acute and Chronic)

As a cough is a symptom of various diseases, these in addition to the cough should be treated.

KINDS OF COUGH: Many writers give several different varieties, but for the sake of convenience I will divide them into two forms, namely: Acute and Chronic.

CAUSE: Acute coughs are generally due to sudden exposure to cold, drafts and are the forerunning symptom of a disease of the organs of breathing.

Chronic Coughs are associated with, and are a result of sore throat, lung fever, pleurisy, bronchitis, catarrh and tuberculosis.

TREATMENT: Under each disease, of which a cough is a symptom, I have also prescribed to include its suppression. The following prescription is reasonable in price, yet very effective in all forms of cough: Tannic Acid, one ounce; Potassi Chlorate, four ounces; Potassi Nitrate, four ounces. Powder well and mix with Black Strap Molasses, one pint, placing container retaining the above in hot water, which assists in dissolving. When this is thoroughly mixed, add Pine Tar, one pint, and place one tablespoonful well back on the tongue with a wooden paddle every three or four hours, according to the severity of the cough.

Sometimes a liniment applied to the throat and windpipe has a good effect, and I would recommend the following on account of its penetrating qualities: Aqua Ammonia Fort., two ounces; Turpentine, two ounces; Raw Linseed Oil, four ounces. Mix and apply twice daily, shaking the contents of the bottle well before using.

COWPOX

(Variola)

CAUSE: Investigations lead us to believe that it is due to a protozoa. So far, the true micro-organism has not been discovered. This disease is very contagious and is transmitted by direct communication but not through the air. Perhaps the most common way of transmitting the disease is by the hands of the milker.

SYMPTOMS: A slight raise in the temperature, especially that of the udder and teats. They are red, swollen and tender and after three or four days small pimples or pustules will appear on the teats about the size of a pea. The pimples or pustules become larger and within a few days may attain the size of one-half inch in diameter. At the end of the second week the pimples or pustules burst and discharge an amber colored fluid leaving raw sores, which cause the animal to suffer intensely when being milked. The supply of milk is also markedly decreased in this condition.

PREVENTION: A person should not milk both healthy and diseased cows unless the hands are thoroughly washed in a Carbolated Solution; the clothes that are likely to come in contact with the udder, coat sleeves, etc., changed.

TREATMENT: It is advisable to give a physic as it has a very good effect on the blood, such as Aloin, two drams, and Ginger, two drams, which is easily prepared and administered by placing in capsule and giving with capsule gun.

Also, the application of Zinc Ointment two or three times a day affords immediate relief and causes the sores to heal rapidly. Good results are also obtained by feeding food that is easily digested, as bran mashes, steamed rolled oats and vegetables.

CUD CHEWING

(Physiology of Rumination)

The cow when eating grass or hay merely moistens it with saliva and swallows, then it passes into the rumen or paunch which acts as a storehouse or reservoir for food. After the paunch or rumen is filled, the cow finds a comfortable place to stand or lie down and she regurgitates it into the mouth by a contraction of the muscles of the walls of the esophagus in small quantities or pellets from the rumen or paunch back into the mouth and is there masticated. When it is chewed finely she swallows and it passes into the second stomach and is there digested for assimilation.

DIARRHOEA

CAUSE: Giving rich succulent foods after being fed on stimulating diets for some time, and such a case may be a benefit to the animal instead of an injury. Turnips, carrots, etc., especially if frozen slightly, are apt to produce it. Also impure and stagnant water which acts as a poison or some irritant in the food, as sand, clay, etc., or it may result from excitement, as driving cattle or shipping cattle in cars when not accustomed to it. Or, it may be the result of an overdose of irritating medicines. Diarrhoea as a rule is not fatal. It is often an effort of nature to relieve some disease, as poison in the blood. The easiest way to get rid of it is by way of the bowels.

SYMPTOMS: It is easily detected. An animal passes large amounts of feces which are of a liquid nature. At first the pulse is but little affected, but after a day or two it becomes weak and slightly increased. If it continues for a few days the pulse increases, the ears and legs get colder than normal, there are slight gripping pains in some cases due to slight irritation or perhaps to slight spasm of the intestines. These pains may increase and result in inflammation of the bowels, especially if the cause is due to stagnant water or irritating drugs.

TREATMENT: In many cases all you have to do is to change the food and clothe the body according to the temperature. Do not let the animal drink large quantities of water at one time. Give pure water in small quantities, but often, and it may be necessary to give medicines. Endeavor to find out the cause and if due to some irritant in the intestines, prepare Flaxseed tea by pouring a quart of boiling water on a half pint of pure Flaxseed, allowing it to cool. Compel the animal to drink it. This is very soothing to the bowels when irritated and also beneficial in removing the irritant; in cases where the

Diarrhoea continues for some time, it is necessary to stop it by administering Gum Catechu, two ounces; Protan, two ounces; Zinc Sulphocarbolates, eight grains. Mix and make into eight capsules and give one capsule every four hours with capsule gun. Keep the animal as quiet as possible and feed non-irritating food that is easily digested, as steamed barley or oats.

DEHORNING

Dehorning is not considered a cruelty as some people hold it, as horns on cattle do not only add discomfort to themselves but add to the owner's risk. It is much better, safer and I think more humane to prevent the growth of horns on calves after they are three or four days old by rubbing the elevations where the horns make their appearance with a pencil of Caustic Potash after being moistened with cold water. Repeat this application two or three times, which is generally sufficient.

When dehorning cattle with clippers or saw, it is well to remove about one-half inch of the flesh of the horn. This gives their head a much better appearance after the horns are removed and healed. When a horn is freshly amputated, apply Oil of Tar occasionally, as it is an antiseptic and prevents infection and the annoyance of flies. However, this should be performed during the season when the flies are less numerous.

DROPSY

(Ascities)

CAUSE: Usually seen in old animals or cattle fed on poor food where the blood becomes so poor, so to speak, that Dropsy follows, The presence of worms frequently stimulates excessive secretions of fluid, producing Dropsy.

SYMPTOMS: The abdomen is abnormally increased in size, flanks are gaunt, paleness of the membranes of the mouth and eyes and a general weakness. Pressure with the hand on the abdominal walls will produce a splashing, watery sound.

TREATMENT: The cause at first should be determined and the disease treated accordingly. If due to worms, withhold all food for twenty-four hours.

Place two ounces of Oil of Turpentine in gelatin capsules and give with capsule gun. Follow this in six hours with two drams of Aloin, three drams of Ginger in gelatin capsule and give with capsule gun. Feed nourishing food as wheat bran mashes and one cup of Flaxseed meal once a day. In their drinking water place one dram of Potassium Iodide two or three times a day. See that this water is drunk and give no other until this is consumed by the animal.

ECZEMA

CAUSE: Insanitary surroundings, as warm, damp stables. Overfeeding, swills, decomposed vegetables. Applying irritating drugs to the skin.

SYMPTOMS: Redness of the skin and the animal rubs itself; is usually confined to a small area at first, but eventually spreads. Considerable inflammation is present, also eruptions of the skin which discharge white, serous, sticky fluid, terminating in scabs and thickness of the skin. Sometimes suppuration or formation of pustules containing pus is present. These symptoms do not always occur in regular succession; in some cases the serums oozing from the skin will be more prominent than in others.

TREATMENT: Determine the cause and remove it. If due to poor food, improve the quality. Also feed laxative food, as hot bran mashes, steamed rolled oats. If the bowels do not act freely, administer Aloin, two drams, and Ginger, three drams. Place in gelatin capsule and give with capsule gun, An ointment made from the following is very effective as an application in this condition: Blue Ointment, one ounce; Zinc Oxide, three ounces. Mix well and apply two or three times a day. A tonic usually has a very good effect in the treatment of this disease, and I would recommend the use of the following: Pulv. Gentian Root, four ounces; Potassium Nitrate, four ounces; Ferri Sulphate, four ounces. Mix and make into twelve capsules and give one capsule two or three times a day with capsule gun.

ERGOT POISON

(Ergotism)

CAUSE: Ergotism is produced by cattle eating fungoid growths which attack kernels and seeds of rye and blue grass, etc. These kernels or seeds grow dark in color and become abnormally large and curved in shape. The infected grass or hay when eaten by cattle contract the arteries, especially those of the legs, just above the feet, although all the arteries in the body are contracted to a certain extent. This disease is frequently seen in Spring and Summer.

SYMPTOMS: Ergot is prescribed in cases of bleeding, because of its contracting effect upon the arteries (closing or stopping the flow of blood) where the blood supply is the weakest, as in the extremities. It is cut off and this, of course, causes the skin just above the hoofs to break or crack as though it were cut with a knife. This shuts off the entire supply of blood to the foot, which mummifies, and the lower portion becomes gangrenous and eventually sloughs off. One of the first effects of Ergot Poison in pregnant cattle is abortion, due to the blood supply to the womb being shut off by its contracting effect on the arteries. Cattle are particularly susceptible to Ergotism.

TREATMENT: When Ergotism is so advanced as to produce sloughing of the feet it is best to destroy the animal. If other animals are affected slightly, find out the cause and remove it. Look to the hay or pasture as the producer. Administer one-half ounce of Chloral Hydrate, two or three times a day in their drinking water or mix it with sufficient quantity of Flaxseed meal to fill an ounce gelatin capsule and give with capsule gun. If the skin is slightly broken above the foot, wash with five per cent solution of Carbolic Acid. Where the feet have become gangrenous amputation of the foot or feet is necessary, which is not advisable unless the animal is very valuable.

FLUKE

(Liver and Lungs)

CAUSE: This disease is contracted by cattle grazing on marshy lands. There are two different species of Fluke that affect the liver and lungs of cattle. They are both flat, leaf-like worms. The Common Liver Fluke is about one-half inch long, while the so-called American Fluke is somewhat larger. In their life history these Flukes depend on snails as intermediate hosts. At a certain stage of development the young Flukes live on snails. They become encysted on stalks and blades of grass which are finally swallowed by grazing cattle.

This disease is most frequently seen in young cattle.

SYMPTOMS: The animal shows no marked signs at first, but eventually the appetite diminishes, rumination or chewing of the cud becomes irregular, the animal becomes dull, hide-bound, hair standing, the visible mucous membranes of the mouth and eyes become pale and bloodless, the eyes discharge watery fluids oozing down the face, temperature varying from two to three degrees above normal and milk supply, if in aged cattle, remarkably reduced. In all cases there is great thirst and the animal becomes very much emaciated and refuses to eat. Swellings about the belly and breast, etc. Diarrhoea at first, alternating with constipation, but finally becomes continuous. The diseased animal succumbs to the malady in from two to six months.

TREATMENT: Medical treatment is unsatisfactory. The disease will be prevented to a considerable extent by giving animals plenty of salt and in the marshes containing pools of water introduce or plant carp, frogs and toads into the infected tracts. These will destroy the young parasites and feed upon the snails which serve as their intermediate hosts. Or, prevent the cattle from grazing upon swampy marshes by fencing them out.

FOOT AND MOUTH DISEASE

(Infectious Aphtha--Epizootica Eczema)

CAUSE: This disease is produced by a specific agent or germ, the exact nature of which is not known. It will pass through the Berkfelt filter, which is the most minute filter known to science, and is therefore known as a filterable virus. This is an eruptive fever and belongs to the class of Exanthematous diseases such as smallpox, measles, scarlet fever, etc. Every outbreak starts from some pre-existing infection. The infection is distributed by manure, pastures, barnyards, hay, drinking troughs, box-cars, ships, boats which have been previously occupied by animals affected with this disease, travel over public highways or man may carry the infection of this disease on his clothing and transmit it to healthy cattle, etc. Foot and Mouth Disease not only affects cattle but attacks a variety of animals, as the horse, sheep, goat, hog, dog, cat, also wild animals as buffalo, deer, antelope, and man himself is not immune from this disease. Children also suffer from Foot and Mouth

Disease, resulting from drinking unboiled milk from infected cattle. Therefore, when purchasing cattle be very careful, as you may be buying an infections disease. Keep the newly purchased animals to themselves for two or three weeks, if possible. This will give ample time for the majority of infectious diseases to develop.

SYMPTOMS: The disease usually makes its first appearance in three to six days after being exposed, by chilling, rise of temperature, and in a day or so pustules varying in size from that of a pin head to that of a pea appear. They appear upon the inner surface of the lips, gums and upper surface of the tongue. The feet also become affected between the digits. The udder usually becomes affected, especially in milking cows. As soon as this disease becomes well established the affected animal evinces great pain when attempting to eat. The animal generally refuses food. In many instances they shut and open the mouth with a smacking sound owing to the stringy saliva flowing from the mouth. The ulcers in the mouth continue to enlarge until they attain the size of one-half to two inches in diameter. The mucous membrane covering these ulcers breaks and a watery discharge escapes. In a few days the surface of the ulcers takes on a whitish appearance. The same changes take place in the feet and the animal becomes very lame and the udder very much swollen, the ulcers discharge, etc.

PREVENTION: When any of the above mentioned symptoms are noticed, non-affected animals should immediately be removed to non-affected quarters. This disease is not communicated through the atmosphere but by the animal coming into direct contact with the infection or virus; hence it is not necessary to move unaffected animals any great distance but merely to clean, sanitary quarters which have not been subjected to any possible infection from the diseased animals. It must be borne in mind that the attendant or helper cannot be too careful in the matter of his own actions and dress as the infection is easily carried through clothes, fecal matter, etc., adhering to shoes or any matter or articles, such as buckets, brushes, rubrags, blankets, etc.

The existence of this disease should at once be reported to your nearest Veterinarian. He will report to the State Veterinarian of your State or to the United States Bureau of Animal Industry at Washington, D. C.

TREATMENT: I cannot recommend any treatment as being satisfactory or a cure, for although under some treatments the animal appears to make a good recovery, in the majority of cases the feet are disfigured and crippled, the udder permanently injured with growths, animal unfit for milking purposes, and the mouth, tongue and teeth left impaired; the mouth and tongue strictured from wounds and the teeth loosened from the gums. Furthermore, should an animal make apparent recovery, it is not immune from a recurrence of the disease. In treating the disease, there is not only danger of spreading the disease to other animals, but to man. The flesh or milk from animals apparently cured should never be used unless first examined by a qualified Veterinarian.

Without question, all animals showing severe symptoms as above described should be at once slaughtered and buried six feet or deeper, covering carcass with Quicklime and then promptly filling grave, according to the Government regulations, which should be followed explicitly. Be careful to disinfect scene of slaughter, as bloodstains, etc. The United States Bureau of Animal Industry regulates the disinfectants to be used and the strength thereof, and as these are subject to change from time to time, I must refer you in this matter to the proper Government authorities.

MEDICAL TREATMENT: If permitted by Government authorities, I would suggest the following treatment as being beneficial: In mild attacks of Foot and Mouth Disease benefits may be derived by cleanliness and the applications of antiseptics as placing Boracic Acid, one dram; Potassium Chlorate, two drams, in a bucket of water, compelling the animal to drink it. Repeat this dose two or three times a day. Also compel the animals to stand in tubs or troughs containing a one in one thousandth solution of Bichloride of Mercury for at least five minutes, twice daily. When other parts of the body become affected, as the cow's udder, apply Carbolated Vaseline twice daily. This treatment should be continued until all ulcers have ceased to discharge. Always keep in mind that this disease is contagious and is transmitted to other animals, as well as to man. For disinfecting corrals, barns, clothing, hands and anything which the diseased animal might come in contact with, I would recommend Coal Tar products, diluted one part to fifty parts warm water. Spray, sprinkle or scrub.

FOOT ROT

(Foul in Foot)

CAUSE: Due to filth or from hard substances accumulating between the two digits, producing irritation and inflammation and suppuration.

SYMPTOMS: Lameness. On examination the foot is swollen, hot and painful to the touch. When the case is of long standing, suppuration occurs and pus will ooze from between the digits, and is very offensive in smell. This condition causes the digits to slough off, if no attempt is made to relieve it.

TREATMENT: Cleanliness. Where there is considerable inflammation present, apply Hot Bran or Flaxseed poultices. Keep clean and treat as an ordinary wound. The following prescription will be found very effective in Foot Rot: Oil of Origanum, four ounces; Oil of Pisis, four ounces; Oil of Turpentine, four ounces. Saturate oakum or cotton with the above liniment placing between the digits and bandage. Feed laxative food, as hot wheat bran mashes and vegetables.

FOUNDER

(Laminitis)

Inflammation of the internal, sensitive structure of the foot.

CAUSE: Overfeeding, overheating, driving on rough, stony soil. Cattle confined to stand on hard floors without exercise frequently suffer from Founder.

SYMPTOMS: The animals lie down a great part of the time. Feet hot and tender and if made to walk they do so with great difficulty. One or all four feet may become affected, although it is more frequently found in the front feet. The temperature is somewhat elevated, varying from 104 to 106 degrees F., breathing very rapid, appetite fairly good and there will be great thirst. Founder in cows reduces the milk secretion, owing to the great fever that is present.

TREATMENT: Apply cold packs to the feet, ice packs preferred. If the animal can be made to stand in a stream of water having a soft bottom, it, perhaps, is the best method of cooling out the feet. Give a physic of Aloin, three drams; Pulv. Gentian Root, two drams. Place in a gelatin capsule and give with capsule gun. To their drinking water add two or three drams of Potassi Nitrate three or four times daily. Animals suffering with Founder should be provided with soft ground to stand on, as their feet will be tender and subject to the chronic form of the disease.

GARGET

(Congestion of the Udder)

CAUSE: Very common in heavy milkers before or just after calving when the bag is very much enlarged and very sensitive; exposure to chilling or standing in drafts or even neglected for too long a time in milking. Injuries may also cause Garget.

SYMPTOMS: The bag is very much enlarged, showing signs of inflammation. The swelling extends well forward following the milk veins. The cow has great difficulty in walking due to sensitiveness of the bag. When milked for two or three days the swelling disappears after the secretion is fully established, but as a rule is tinged with blood. Sometimes small clots of milk or cheese-like particles are ejected with the milk.

TREATMENT: Give a physic consisting of Aloin, two drams; Pulv. Ginger, three drams. Place in gelatin capsule and give with capsule gun: Hyposulphite of Soda, sixteen ounces; Nitrate of Potassi, four ounces. Mix and make into sixteen powders. Give one powder three times a day in drinking water or place in gelatin capsule and give with capsule gun. Also dissolve Bichloride of Mercury, two grains; Boracic Acid, two drams, in one quart of boiling hot water. When this solution cools to about blood temperature, after stripping all milk fluid or pus from the affected teat or teats, inject with an ordinary bulb injection syringe after placing a teat tube into the end from which the air escapes when the bulb is pressed. Now, place the end of the syringe retaining the teat tube in the affected teat, the other end place in a bottle or vessel containing the solution and gently press the bulb and inject about a pint of the solution in each affected quarter. Leave the solution in the teat for only fifteen to twenty minutes and milk out thoroughly. Repeat this treatment two or three times a day.

For an external application the following ointment has given remarkably good results: Blue Ointment and Zinc Ointment, equal parts. Mix well and apply two or three times daily.

HARD MILKERS

CAUSE: A thickness or contraction of the mucous membranes lining the teat or growths inside the teat.

TREATMENT: All antiseptic precautions should be carried out in this operation, as boiling the instruments and then covering them with Carbolated Vaseline. Then with a hidden bistoury or a knife concealed in a tube, force upward into the teat, then press out the little blade and draw the instrument down the teat, making about four incisions equal distance apart around the inner surface of the teat. The use of self-retaining teat dilators prevents the contraction of the cut surface, permitting them to remain in the teat for two weeks, removing them only when the milk is being stripped from the teat. Always place them in boiling water and cover with Carbolated Vaseline before inserting.

HOLLOW HORN

Horns of the cattle tribe are normally hollow, although a core extends well into the horn. This, however, is merely a prolongation of a porous bone of the head which affords a point for the horns' attachment, consequently when a cow is sick and the temperature is elevated, the horns are naturally hot, it being the symptom of a disease and not a disease of itself, and which should be treated under its special heading.

The supposed disease "Hollow Horn" once upon a time was treated by boring a hole into the horn with a small gimlet and pouring Turpentine into the opening. This treatment is useless and harmful. It produces inflammation of the frontal sinuses of the head and chances are death of the animal will follow as a result of the treatment and not of the disease.

INDIGESTION

CAUSE: Animals with a voracious appetite will overload their stomachs with food that is hard to digest or is decomposed, causing the organs of assimilation to become weakened, sluggish and incapable of doing their proper work.

SYMPTOMS: The animal ceases to ruminate (chew its cud); stands quietly, hair rough, nose dry, temperature elevated one to two degrees, breathing usually faster than normal with slight grunts at each expiration of air from the lungs. The secretions of milk are suddenly diminished. If the hand is placed against the left side and quickly removed, a marked depression or pit will remain, which shows that the paunch is full of undigested food. Bloating is also frequently accompanied by indigestion.

TREATMENT: Administer Aloin, three drams; Ginger, three drams. Place in capsule and give with capsule gun. Permit the animal to drink all the water possible. If bloating is present give two-ounce capsules filled with Turpentine with capsule gun. A tonic is quite necessary in this condition, and the following I am sure will be followed by good results if the case is not of too long a standing: Sodium Bicarbonate, eight ounces; Pulv. Nux Vomica, four ounces; Pulv. Gentian Root, four ounces; Pulv. Ginger, four ounces. Place two tablespoonfuls in gelatin capsule and give with capsule gun every six hours. Very good results are also obtained from rectal injections of soap and warm water. Feed good nourishing food sparingly, compelling the animal to exercise, etc.

INFLAMMATION OF THE BAG

(Simple Mammitis)

CAUSE: Injuries, as blows, kicks, etc.; lying on cold, rough ground or floor, standing in drafts, sudden change of weather. Derangement of the system is likely to affect the udder; poorly milked or stripped cows are often victims of Mammitis. Infections in the teat from inserting dirty instruments, as using a bicycle pump for the treatment of Milk Fever. Cows with a retained afterbirth are likely to infect the udder by switching their tail. This condition is very common in heavy milkers following calving.

SYMPTOMS: The animal chills, hair stands, temperature elevated from one to three degrees above normal; ears, horns and legs cold, which may suddenly become very hot; pulse rapid, breathing hurried, bag hard and swollen and very tender on pressure. When attempts are made to milk, a watery substance comes away, almost colorless at first, but later becomes tinged with blood and pus and has a fetid odor. The cow's muzzle is dry, appetite poor, but great thirst exists. This condition may affect one or more quarters of the udder. Abscesses may form and the udder break and a thick yellowish pus oozes out or the milk glands may solidify and cause hard, lumpy growths in the udder.

TREATMENT: Prevention. If an animal is once slightly affected with inflammation of the bag, it is likely to develop a bad case of Mammitis from the slightest injury or exposure as stated above, which depreciates a cow considerably as a milk producer, especially on the market. Great care should be exercised when purchasing a cow for milking purposes. See that the teats and udder are sound, free from lumps, etc.

MEDICAL TREATMENT: Hyposulphite of Soda, sixteen ounces; Nitrate of Potassi, four ounces. Mix and make into sixteen powders. Give one powder three times a day in drinking water or place in a gelatin capsule and give with a capsule gun. Also, dissolve Bichloride of Mercury, two grains; Boracic Acid, two drams, in one quart of boiling hot water. When this solution cools to about blood temperature, after stripping all milk fluid or pus from the affected teat or teats, inject with an ordinary bulb injection syringe after placing a teat tube into the end from which the air escapes when the bulb is pressed. Now, place this end of the syringe retaining the teat tube in the affected teat; the other end place in a bottle or vessel containing the solution and gently press the bulb and inject about a pint of the solution into each affected quarter. Leave the solution in the teat for only fifteen to twenty minutes and milk out thoroughly. Repeat this treatment two or three times a day.

For an external application, the following ointment has given remarkably good results: Blue Ointment, two ounces; Lard, two ounces. Mix well and apply twice daily.

INFLAMMATION OF THE EYE

(Conjunctivitis)

CAUSE: Injuries; irritating gases, from an animal standing in dark and poorly ventilated stables or foreign bodies in the eye, as chaff, etc.

SYMPTOMS: A constant flow of tears from the eye running down the animal's face, which are due to the inflammation of the lining membranes of the eye. The eye is partially or completely closed.

TREATMENT: If due to a foreign body, remove it. In order to accomplish this, the animal must be placed in a stanchion, the head twisted and the eyelid turned back. Do not use burned alum as this will only make the condition worse. Use Boracic Acid, thirty grains; distilled water, one ounce. Apply to the eye three or four times daily, using an ordinary eye-dropper.

INFLAMMATION OF THE HEART SACK

(Pericarditis)

CAUSE: Cattle being ruminants, therefore, not masticating their food finely before swallowing, consequently foreign bodies, such as nails, wire, etc., are picked up with the food and taken into the rumen or paunch. These sharp objects penetrate the walls of the paunch, rumen or first stomach and pierce the membrane or sack surrounding the heart, which produces an inflammation of the heart sack, or Pericarditis.

SYMPTOMS: Symptoms develop very slowly or indications of indigestion will be present as the appetite is variable, temperature elevated, breathing labored, the animal avoids walking down hill as it causes pain from the stomach and intestines pressing the lungs against the heart. The symptoms, however, are so slight that they may easily escape the notice of a casual observer. The animal eventually becomes poor, emaciated and dies. If you open the heart sack, it will be found full of watery pus.

TREATMENT: Unsuccessful, as this disease is seldom diagnosed correctly, and if it is an operation is necessary and this does not prove successful in the majority of cases.

INFLAMMATION OF THE KIDNEYS

CAUSE: Injuries in the region of the kidneys, exposure to cold weather, especially in cows soon after calving. Eating poisonous plants, decomposed food or drinking stagnant water, irritating medicines given ignorantly of their bad effects are frequently followed by inflammation of the kidneys.

SYMPTOMS: The attack will first be noticed by slight shivering or chilling followed by an increased temperature, breathing increased. The animal attempts to urinate frequently and the amount passed is small and of a dark amber color and may be flaked with blood. There will be stiffness and straddling of the hind legs which is always present during urinary disorders. There may be slight swelling and tenderness over the kidneys. As the disease progresses the animal grows weak and finally dies if prompt relief is not afforded. Fortunately this disease is not common among cattle.

TREATMENT: Clothe the animal if the weather is cold. Mild physics are beneficial, as Aloin, one and one-half drams; Ginger, two drams; Nux Vomica, two drams, placed in a gelatin capsule and given with capsule gun. Also, the following, which is very soothing to the urinary tract: Potassium Acetate, Potassium Bromide, each four ounces, made into sixteen powders. Give one powder every four hours in their drinking water. Feed nitrogenous food as hot wheat bran mashes, steamed rolled oats, and see that the animal has pure water to drink.

INFLAMMATION OF THE PENIS

CAUSE: Injuries received from snags, walking through the underbrush, jumping fences, etc.

SYMPTOMS: Arched back, swelling of the sheath and in some cases a discharge. It may be serious enough to affect the appetite and cause fever.

TREATMENT: Wash out the sheath two or three times daily with a three per cent solution of Boracic Acid. If the inflammation extends pretty well back in the sheath, it is advisable to inject this solution with a syringe, carefully, as far back as possible. Withdraw the syringe, holding the opening of the sheath so as to retain the solution for a few minutes before allowing it to escape.

Feed laxative food and supply the animal with fresh water to drink. If there is considerable fever, administer Potassium Nitrate, Pulv. Nux Vomica, each two ounces. Make into eight capsules and give one capsule two or three times a day.

INFLAMMATION OF THE WOMB

CAUSE: Injuries, as bruises, laceration, sustained during calving, especially where the cow is assisted with instruments or hands that are not thoroughly aseptic, an animal retaining the afterbirth which undergoes putrefaction, and consequently sets up an inflammation of the womb, or perhaps the animal may become infected during the act of removing the afterbirth if the operator is neglectful about washing his hands or washing the womb out thoroughly.

SYMPTOMS: The animal will chill, the temperature elevated two or three degrees, the back will be arched, stiffness of the hind parts, legs, ears and horns cold, nose hot and dry, grinding of the teeth, the cow usually remains standing, ceases to chew her cud, the secretions of milk will be markedly reduced and a day or so after the symptoms appear, there will be a discharge from the womb of a reddish lumpy nature. This becomes thick and yellow containing small particles of flesh, showing that the inner lining of the womb is sloughing. This discharge is very offensive in odor. A cow in this condition requires the best of care or she will die as the decomposed substance in the womb may be absorbed into the circulation and produce Pyemia or Septicemia (Blood Poison).

TREATMENT: Give Aloin, two drams; Pulv. Ginger, three drams, place in a gelatin capsule and give with capsule gun. Flush out the womb thoroughly with a tablespoonful of Carbolic Acid to one gallon of water two or three times a day. A convenient instrument for flushing out the womb can be made from an ordinary funnel and a clean hose about four feet long. This answers the purpose of an injection syringe very well. In their drinking water add the following: Hyposulphite of Soda, sixteen ounces; Potassium Iodide, two ounces. Make into sixteen powders and give one powder two or three times a day.

In addition to the above treatment it is necessary to give alteratives and bitter tonics to build up the condition of the animal as soon as possible. The following will be found very effective: Pulv. Gentian Root, four ounces; Pulv. Ferri Sulphate, four ounces; Nitrate of Potash, four ounces. Mix and make into sixteen powders and give one powder three times a day. Place in a gelatin capsule and administer with a capsule gun.

My reasons for giving animals medicine in capsules are:

1. There is no danger of liquids, as in drenching, escaping into the lungs.

2. Any drug having any beneficial effects as a tonic is very bitter, consequently the only way the animal will take it is by placing in capsule.

JOINT ILL, NAVEL ILL

(Umbilical Pyemia and Septicemia)

CAUSE: This disease is produced by various germs entering the navel cord of newly born calves when dropped, the navel being freshly severed and its coming in contact with filth and manure where germs are numerous, consequently germs adhere and enter the blood stream. Calf Scours as a rule is associated with this disease.

SYMPTOMS: Swelling of the joints which are very hot and painful on pressure, and when the calf is made to move it walks stiffly and slowly, does not care to nurse its mother or take any food, temperature elevated from 105 to 108 degrees F., breathing hurried, pulse very weak and quick. There will be an offensive discharge from the navel cord of a yellowish color and swollen joints finally break and also discharge a thick yellow pus. The calf becomes emaciated and finally dies from exhaustion.

TREATMENT: Prevention. Provide clean surroundings for cows when calving, and in addition to this have a one in one-thousandth solution of Bichloride of Mercury on hand. Wash the navel well in the solution once a day until the cord is thoroughly dried.

MEDICAL TREATMENT: Unsuccessful. Sometimes the calf recovers, but at best the calf is badly stunted and is very seldom worth keeping. However, the following method of treatment has been followed with fairly good results: Wash the navel cord well in a one-thousandth solution of Bichloride of Mercury two or three times a day and give Zinc Sulphocarbolates, one-fourth grain; Potassi Iodide, five grains, in a little water or milk three or four times a day. Feed them three or four eggs a day, molasses, fresh milk. This will keep up the strength and vitality and a good recovery may follow, although it is an exception and not a rule.

LACERATION OF THE EYELID

CAUSE: An eyelid may be torn on the manger, rubbing post or barb wire fence, etc.

TREATMENT: Wash the lacerated portions of the eye thoroughly with a five per cent solution of Carbolic Acid. It may be necessary to take a few stitches in the wound or the torn edges may be cut off with a pair of sharp scissors. If stitches have been taken, they should be removed after the parts have united and the eye kept clean. A very convenient application for the eye in this condition is Boracic Acid, one dram; Distilled Water, four ounces. Apply liberally to the eye.

LEECHES

(Blood Suckers)

Leeches which suck blood of cattle are sometimes taken up by the animals when drinking water from ponds, etc. The leeches attach themselves to the inner surface of the mouth or nose, and sometimes reach the upper part of windpipe or the gullet. Bleeding at the mouth or nose may be noticed, the membranes where the leeches attach themselves become congested and swollen, and as a result of the loss of blood anemic condition follows.

TREATMENT: If the leeches can be reached, they are easily destroyed by cutting them in two with a pair of scissors or they may be removed with a pair of forceps or with the fingers after wrapping a piece of cloth around them so as to prevent slipping.

Steam from boiling hot water containing Pine Tar or Oil of Turpentine may cause leeches to release their hold if they cannot be removed by other means. In ponds where leeches are numerous, eels should be introduced as they feed upon blood suckers of this species.

LUMPY JAW

(Wooden Tongue, Big Head, Actinomycosis)

CAUSE: The Ray Fungus. This organism which occurs in the tissues in the form of russets is directly transmitted from one animal to another. It seems apparent that the fungus is conveyed into the tissues of the mouth by various food stuff through slight wounds of the mucous membranes of the mouth or an animal that has decayed teeth or during the shedding of milk teeth. The Ray Fungus is found naturally vegetated or clinging on the awns of barley, the spears of oats and on other grains. Quantities of fungi have been found between the vegetable fibers of barley which had penetrated the gums of cattle and on the awns of grain imbedded in their tongues.

Lumpy Jaw can also be transmitted by coming in contact with or eating food over which lumpy jawed cattle have slobbered. A healthy animal eating such food with very slight bruises or abrasions of the mouth will contract the disease very readily. This disease is misleading as other organs are affected with the Ray Fungi or the Bacillus of Actinomycosis, as the lungs and even the digestive organs have been found to be affected with this disease.

SYMPTOMS: External symptoms or signs are the only means by which to ascertain the disease. Its exact location is on the lower jaw bone near its angle. It may also affect the upper jaw, but this is an exception and not a rule. Internally it may affect the tongue, mouth, throat or lungs, but rarely the intestines. This enlargement continues to grow until it reaches the size of that of a man's head, breaks and discharges pus. The animal becomes poor and emaciated, the hair takes on a dull, roughened appearance and in many cases it is very difficult for it to eat, especially where the disease separates the gums and bone from the teeth and causes them to become very loose or to drop out. The animal in the latter stages of this disease generally dies from starvation.

TREATMENT: Successful in its first stages. Soft, nitrogenous food should be fed, such as wheat bran mashes, steamed rolled oats or barley, hay dampened with clean water, so as to make it pliable. Hay containing woody matter as stems, etc., should not be fed to an animal affected with Lumpy Jaw as it tends to aggravate the disease. Internally in their drinking water give two drams of Potassium Iodide morning and night. This treatment, however, should be omitted when the animal's skin becomes scaly or when an excessive watery discharge flows from the eyes. On the outer surface over the enlargement apply the following ointment: Red Iodide of Mercury, four drams; Lard, two ounces. Mix well and rub in briskly for twenty minutes every five or six days for three weeks. The cure can generally be ascertained by the animal gaining in flesh, although the lump may remain. Where Lumpy Jaw is of long standing so as to impair the use of the animal's tongue or teeth, it is best to destroy the animal, as this lessens the possibilities of infecting healthy animals.

LUNG FEVER

(Pneumonia)

CAUSE: Generally follows congestion of the lungs. It may be due to parasitic organisms or exposure to cold, drafts when warm after being driven, etc. Drenching perhaps is the most common cause as it is very difficult for a cow to swallow when the head is elevated; inhaling smoke, gases, etc., also tend to produce pneumonia.

SYMPTOMS: Chilling or shivering, temperature elevated to 105 or 106 degrees F., nose hot and dry, horns and legs cold. Pulse rapid though strong, breathing fast and the appetite very good in some cases. The animal urinates small quantities of urine but often, of a dark amber color. A discharge from the nose follows, also a cough. If the ear is placed back of the fore leg, a dry crackling sound can be heard something on the order of rubbing hair between the fingers.

TREATMENT: Place the animal in a dry, well lighted and ventilated stable, but avoid drafts. Give Pulv. Iodide of Ammonia, one ounce; Pulv. Potassium Nitrate, four ounces; Pulv. Nux Vomica, four ounces; Pulv. Capsicum, one ounce; Quinine, one ounce. Mix well and make into thirty-two powders. Place one powder in gelatin capsule and administer every three or four hours with capsule gun. Supply the animal with fresh water at all times. Feed laxative food as hot wheat bran mashes or steamed rolled oats. Also feed vegetables, such as potatoes, apples, carrots and kale. It is also advisable to apply the following over the region of the lungs just back of the fore legs: Aqua Ammonia Fort., four ounces; Oil of Turpentine, four ounces; Raw Linseed Oil, six ounces. Mix and shake well and apply two or three times daily. It is also advisable to hand rub the legs and bandage them with woolen cloths. If the above treatment is properly carried out, the animal will make a complete recovery in a week or ten days.

LOSS OF CUD

CAUSE: This condition cannot always be traced to a definite cause, as it is a symptom of all diseases where the process of rumination is interfered with. The only method by which a cow will again chew her cud is to restore her back to health by the proper medical treatment. Artificial cuds are of no value and frequently are a detriment to the animal. Other symptoms aside from those of the animal not chewing cud will always make their appearance, as constipation, diarrhoea, elevation of the temperature, etc. The animal should be thoroughly examined and the disease treated under its special heading.

MANGE

(Scabies)

CAUSE: There are four different parasites which produce Mange or Scabies in cattle. However, three of these parasites are rarely seen. The Symbotis Communis is the parasite commonly seen in American cattle. These parasites multiply very rapidly and are conveyed from diseased animals to healthy ones by their bodies coming in contact with one another and by healthy animals rubbing against fences, walls, posts, etc., where mangy cattle have previously rubbed.

SYMPTOMS: Scabs, loss of hair, intense itching, the animals are constantly rubbing or licking themselves. The parts showing the first signs of Mange are those about the croup, or the root of the tail, the neck and withers, but as the disease progresses and no attempts are offered for its eradication, it finally spreads and covers the entire body. The scabs become ulcerated, the animal becomes weakened, emaciated and eventually dies.

TREATMENT: Dipping in wood or concrete vats is the most satisfactory method of treating Mange. The regular lime and sulphur dip as recommended by the United States Bureau of Animal Industry is inexpensive and effective.

MEASLY BEEF

Is produced by a larva of common tapeworm of man. These small tapeworm cysts (taenia saginata) are about the size of a pea and found in the flesh of cattle, which become infected by eating food or drinking water which has been contaminated by the feces of persons harboring adult tapeworms. Then again, the person becomes infected by eating raw or rare flesh of cattle infected with the larva stage of Measly Beef. Great care should be exercised to prevent cattle from becoming infected with this parasite. Persons' feces should not be placed where it will infect food or drinking water that is consumed by cattle.

MILK FEVER

(Parturient Apoplexy)

CAUSE: Certain conditions predispose cows to Milk Fever, as being heavy milk producers, cows having enormous digestive power and being heavily fed on nitrogenous food naturally are in a good condition, consequently at the time of calving, or shortly after, they are likely to develop a case of Milk Fever, It is more common during summer months, although this condition may develop at any time of the year in the type of cow described above.

SYMPTOMS: At or a few days after calving, the cow is noticed hanging back in the stall, dull, languid, with an unsteady movement of the hind legs. If the cow is made to walk, she steps unsteadily or staggers, pays no attention to her calf; she finally becomes so paralyzed that she falls and is unable to rise. The pupils of the eyes are dilated and the membranes reddened or congested with blood. The cow may lie on her breast or flat on her side, but most likely upon her breast and her head turned in the region of the flank. She apparently is sound asleep. If the eyeball is touched with the fingers she does not close the eye, nor will she evince any pain when being pricked with a pin on any part of the body. The nose is dry, the temperature is below normal in most cases. Just how the name of this disease started by the name of "Milk Fever" I cannot understand.

TREATMENT: When the above signs are noticed, whether the cow is standing or lying down in a paralyzed condition, obtain an ordinary bulb injection syringe; insert a tube in the end from which the air escapes. After washing both syringe and teat tube in a five per cent solution of Carbolic Acid, milk or strip out all the milk possible from the bag, then insert the teat tube that is connected to the syringe in each teat, filling them well with air, and repeat this treatment every hour until the cow stops staggering, or if lying down, stands on her feet. It is necessary to strip the milk from the bag before giving an injection of air. If the cow is lying flat on her side, prop her up by placing bags of hay or straw against her side, also make her as comfortable as possible. If lying in the hot sun, provide shade by placing a canopy over her made from burlap; if the weather is chilly, blanket; if flies annoy her, use some fly repellant.

This disease is satisfactorily treated. Where ninety per cent of the cows died at one time, ninety per cent can be saved by the above treatment. It is a custom with some people to use an ordinary bicycle pump for treatment of Milk Fever. This should not be practiced, as there is great danger of infecting the bag and producing serious complications.

MEDICAL OR AFTER TREATMENT: Never drench a cow. Give a physic consisting of Aloin, two drams; Ginger, three drams. Place in a gelatin capsule and give with a capsule gun. Also, give tonics as Pulv. Gentian Root, two ounces; Pulv. Capsicum, one ounce; Pulv. Nux Vomica, two ounces. Mix and place into eight gelatin capsules. Give one capsule every eight hours. This tonic is quite necessary, as it stimulates their appetite, braces up their nervous system and prevents any complications that might otherwise follow.

PARALYSIS

(Congestion of the Brain or Spinal Cord)

CAUSE: May be due to a morbid condition of the brain or spinal cord, concussion of the spinal cord, fractures of the bones of the spinal column, or violent shocks or jars of the brain, or pressure due to fractures of the skull, or dilated or ruptured blood vessels. Paralysis also occurs in poorly fed, weak cows when exposed to cold or wet weather during the latter stages of pregnancy. Sometimes the back portion of the bowels (the rectum) becomes paralyzed so as to interfere with the expulsion of the feces which becomes dry and more or less impacted. This condition may also occur in connection with Ergot, Forage or Lead Poisoning, Milk Fever or Parturient Apoplexy.

SYMPTOMS: Appear very suddenly. The animal is unable to stand, lies quietly and groans occasionally. Constipation generally accompanies this condition. Sometimes great pain is present, especially if due to fracture or pressure, as above mentioned.

TREATMENT: If just due to weakness; exposure to cold, wet weather; cows prior to calving; slight injuries or mild effect of poisons, it is successfully treated by placing the animal in a comfortable, well lighted stall, omitting drafts, feeding nourishing food, as warm wheat bran mashes, steamed rolled oats or barley and linseed meal; tea to drink prepared as follows: Pour one quart of boiling water on one-half pint of Pure Flaxseed, allowing it to cool, and compel the animal to drink it. Repeat this once or twice daily, especially if the animal is pregnant. A physic consisting of Aloin, two drams; Ginger, two drams; prepared in capsule and given with a capsule gun is very effective, but this, however, should not be administered to heavily pregnant cows. Endeavor to move their bowels by careful feeding of laxative food and rectal injections of soap and water. Nerve stimulants are necessary and I have derived good results from the following: Pulv. Nux Vomica, four ounces; Pulv. Ginger, four ounces; Pulv. Gentian Root, four ounces. Make into sixteen capsules and give one capsule every four or six hours. Also apply powdered mustard, moistened with a sufficient quantity of water to make a paste, and rub over the full length of the spine about eight inches in width. This should be covered with paper which will adhere readily to the mustard and water. This application can be repeated every twenty-four hours until satisfactory results have been obtained.

RED WATER

(Hematuria)

CAUSE: Marshy pastures, water from rich decomposed soil. Vegetation also has a tendency to produce it as cattle eating green shoots from oak, ash, hellebore, hazel and other resinous plants, etc.

SYMPTOMS: Bloody urine containing no blood clots. This condition is not noticed as a general rule until the cow loses flesh and the production of milk is considerably decreased. One particular symptom of this disease is the milk being exceptionally foamy and perhaps tinged with blood. If the disease is left to run its course, the cow will become emaciated and eventually dies.

TREATMENT: Find out the cause and remove it if possible. See that the water supply is clean, feed nitrogenous food, as wheat bran mashes or steamed rolled oats. Do not permit the animal to eat resinous plants as stated above.

Administer Pulv. Gentian Root, four ounces; Pulv. Nux Vomica, four ounces; Pulv. Ferri Sulphate, four ounces. Mix and make into sixteen capsules and give one capsule two or three times a day with capsule gun. If the animal is constipated, give two drams of Aloin, three drams of Ginger. Place in capsule and give with capsule gun.

RETAINED AFTERBIRTH

CAUSE: Retained afterbirth may follow normal or abnormal calving where there has been more or less inflammation of the womb prior to giving birth, which causes the afterbirth to adhere firmly to its attachments. Cows in poor condition fed on poor food during cold weather are very susceptible to this accident; also very common in aged cows.

SYMPTOMS: Very easily detected by portions of the membranes (afterbirth) protruding from the Womb or Vulva, which becomes decomposed very shortly and offensive in odor. This accident is very serious when absorption is produced, ill health, drying up of the milk in addition to producing inflammation of the womb, Whites, etc. It may produce blood-poisoning and chances are you will lose your animal.

PREVENTION: Very important. Feed the cow on food that is easily digested and supply her with fresh water to drink that is not too cold. Flaxseed Tea is very beneficial if given a day or so prior to calving and is prepared by pouring a quart of boiling hot water on one-half pint of Flaxseed, permitting it to cool of its own accord. Then compel the animal to drink it. This appears to have a very good effect on separating the afterbirth from the mushroom-like bodies of the womb to which it is attached.

MEDICAL TREATMENT: The afterbirth should not be pulled away by force, as it may tear, leaving small portions unremoved that perhaps would result in Inflammation of the Womb or Whites. To remove the afterbirth insert the hand and carefully detach it from its attachments, being very careful that the cotyledons are not torn off. After this has been carefully removed, wash out the womb with Carbolic Acid solution about two and one-half per cent. An instrument can be made for this purpose very easily from a clean piece of hose about four feet long and an ordinary funnel. Sometimes it is necessary to give physics, as Aloin, two drams; Ginger, two drams. Place in a gelatin capsule and give with capsule gun.

In addition to the above, stimulants are also advisable such as powdered Nux Vomica, powdered Capsicum, powdered Ginger, powdered Nitrate of Potash, equal parts four ounces. Make twenty-four capsules and give one capsule three times a day.

RHEUMATISM

CAUSE: Exposure, especially when the animal is permitted to lie on cold damp soils or floors. Another common cause is an animal exposed to cold drafts after perspiring or weakened after severe physical exercise.

SYMPTOMS: Stiffness when walking, variable appetite, constipation, hair unthrifty looking. Passage of urine is scant and of an amber color, usually slight elevation in temperature and the animal lies down a great part of the time. There are two forms of rheumatism--muscular and articular. The former affects the muscles of the body, while the latter affects the joints. There will be swellings that are tender on pressure, which may shift to different parts of the body.

TREATMENT: Place the animal in warm dry quarters with a sufficient quantity of clean bedding. Feed foods that are easily digested, as wheat bran mashes and steamed rolled oats and vegetables. Keep pure, cold water within the animal's reach at all times. The following prescription has been found very effective in the treatment of this disease: Sodium Salicylate, six ounces; Nux Vomica, two ounces; Pulv. Gentian Root, two ounces; Nitrate of Potash, two ounces. Mix and make into sixteen capsules and give one capsule three times daily with capsule gun. If the bowels are constipated give Aloin, two drams; Ginger, three drams. Place in capsule and give with capsule gun. When the joints or muscles become swollen and inflamed, the following liniment will be found very effective in reducing the swellings: Aqua Ammonia Fort., two ounces; Oil of Turpentine, three ounces; Sweet Oil, six ounces. Mix and apply by rubbing in well two or three times a day.

RINGWORM

CAUSE: Due to a vegetable parasite. It affects the hair and the outer layer of skin and is highly contagious, being transmitted from one animal to another.

SYMPTOMS: The disease usually appears in the form of circular patches of the skin, which soon become denude of hair. Sometimes a white sticky discharge and the formation of scaly, brittle crusts on the patches appear, silvery gray in color. They are generally confined to the head and neck. It is a common disease among young cattle in the Winter and Spring. This disease is attended with more or less itching and is communicable to man.

TREATMENT: Remove the scabs or crusts with soap and warm water. However, the surface of the body should be well dried after washing each time. Apply Tincture of Iodine with a camel-hair brush to the spots denuded of hair. It is quite necessary that the barn and rubbing posts be disinfected by spraying or washing them with a twenty-five per cent solution of Carbolic Acid.

ROUND WORM

CAUSE: An animal swallowing the eggs of the parasite in food or water which has been contaminated with the feces of infected cattle. There are two species, the large Roundworm measuring from five to fourteen inches in length, the other small Roundworm varying in size from one-quarter of an inch to two inches in length. Both the small and large Roundworms infest the intestines of cattle and calves. These worms, especially small Roundworms, irritate the mucous lining of the intestines, which may cause severe inflammation.

SYMPTOMS: Anemia, appetite variable, diarrhoea, general weakness, dullness and excessive thirst; also a paleness of the visible membranes of the mouth, nose and eye. Worms frequently pass with the feces and can be readily seen by a close observer.

PREVENTIVE TREATMENT: See prevention of Twisted Stomach Worm.

MEDICAL TREATMENT: Withhold all food from eighteen to twenty-four hours. To calves, two to eight months old, give two teaspoonfuls of Turpentine in a pint of milk; to yearlings, give one tablespoonful. Place in gelatin capsule and give with capsule gun. To cattle one year old and over place one ounce in a gelatin capsule and give with capsule gun. This treatment is to be repeated twice during the intervals of ten days or two weeks, which insures the expulsion of the eggs of worms that escaped the first treatment. Also keep salt where cattle can lick it frequently.

RUPTURE

(Abdominal Hernia)

CAUSE: This disease occasionally occurs in calves by receiving blows from the cow's horns on the right flank. After such an accident a swelling forms near the last ribs. This swelling may be either hot and painful or soft to the touch. It can be made to disappear by careful pressure when the sides of the rupture through which it has passed can be felt. On removing the pressure the rupture soon regains its swollen appearance. Similar conditions may also occur in aged cattle, usually due to injuries, such as being kicked by a horse, etc., or due to a weakness of the muscles that are ruptured sometimes during difficult birth.

TREATMENT: Feed the animal on laxative food and feed sparingly on bulky food such as hay, straw and grass. Round the edges of a block of wood a little smaller, but the same shape as the rupture. After wrapping with cloth nicely, place it over the rupture, then place around the body. This permits the ruptured muscles to grow together, providing the animal is properly dieted as stated above.

Sometimes a rupture of long standing or a newly produced rupture may be treated by injecting strong solutions of Common Salt around the torn edges of the muscles. This causes swelling and inflammation, which respectively forces the protruded intestines back and closes the opening. There is some danger attached to this method of treatment, and if attempted I would advise the services of a competent Veterinarian.

SCUM OVER THE EYE

CAUSE: See Inflammation of the Eye.

SYMPTOMS: The eye has a smoke-colored appearance.

TREATMENT: Silver Nitrate, two grains, thoroughly dissolved in one ounce of Distilled Water, Apply with dropper two or three times a day. Feed the animal on food that is easily digested and confine the animal to a cool, clean, dark stall.

SORE THROAT

(Laryngitis and Pharyngitis)

CAUSE: Sudden cooling of the surface of the body, as when cattle are exposed to cold weather or cold rain or the inhaling of irritating gases.

SYMPTOMS: The muzzle is dry, temperature slightly elevated and saliva dribbles from the corners of the mouth. The animal either does not swallow, or swallows with great difficulty, and holds its head in a stiff, straight position, moving it as little as possible. The eyelids are half-closed and bloodshot, and the animal occasionally grinds the teeth. After masticating the food the animal drops it out of its mouth as if to avoid the pain of swallowing, and also evinces great pain when pressure is applied from the outside. In acute attacks of sore throat, the animal coughs with great difficulty and breathes very noisily. The nostrils are dilated and nose extended.

TREATMENT: Place the animal in as comfortable a place as possible, permitting as much fresh air as possible, but avoiding drafts. Blanket the animal if the weather is chilly, also hand rub the legs and bandage with woolen cloths.

Administer Chlorate of Potash, two ounces; Nitrate of Potash, two ounces; Tannic Acid, one-half ounce; Molasses, eight ounces. Mix well and place one tablespoonful on the tongue every three or four hours. Feed soft food, as wheat bran mashes and steamed rolled oats, or boiled vegetables. Give drinking water with the chill taken off.

It is always necessary to apply liniments to the throat, and I would advise the application of Aqua Ammonia Fort., four ounces; Oil of Turpentine, four ounces, and Sweet Oil, four ounces. Apply and rub in well two or three times a day.

STRINGY MILK

CAUSE: Cows wading or standing in stagnant pools of water. Frequently stringy milk results from fungi entering the udder. This takes on an infectious form, and several cows may become affected at one time.

SYMPTOMS: Although the milk appears perfectly normal when first milked, it becomes stringy after being let stand for a few hours. If a needle is inserted in the milk and slowly withdrawn, the milk will adhere to the point and have a stringy appearance. If the cow is examined carefully, the temperature will be found to be elevated a degree or two, the appetite poor and the nose dry.

TREATMENT: Feed laxative food and see that they have fresh water to drink. Also, place two drams of Soda Bisulphite once or twice a day in gelatin capsule and give with capsule gun. Do not permit the cow to come in contact with stagnant pools of water that carry this infection. Perhaps the best plan is to fence out all such stagnant pools of water.

SUPPRESSION OF MILK

(Absence of Milk)

CAUSE: Unusually due to poor health, debility, emaciated, chronic diseases of the bag, or wasting of its glands from various diseases or impure food. Sometimes this condition is produced without any apparent cause.

TREATMENT: Determine the cause, if possible, and remove it. Feed warm wheat bran mashes, steamed rolled oats or barley. Administer Pulv. Anise Seed, one-half ounce, two or three times a day. This has a very good effect in this particular condition. Also rub the bag and strip the teats often, and apply Oil of Lavender. The majority of cases respond to this treatment if not due to chronic disease of the bag.

TAPEWORM

CAUSE: Small portions of tapeworms, consisting of one or more segments, are occasionally seen in the droppings of infected cattle. The infection is undoubtedly taken in with the food or water, infection being spread by the eggs of the parasite, and being expelled with the feces of an infected animal. The eggs being swallowed by insects, worms or snails, which act as an intermediate host, and which when swallowed accidentally by cattle while grazing or drinking carry with them into the animal's stomach the infectious stage of the tapeworm. Aged cattle do not seem to suffer much from tapeworms, but in calves these parasites cause scours and rapid emaciation.

SYMPTOMS: Emaciation, diarrhoea, loss of flesh, ravenous appetite, paleness of the mucous membranes of the mouth and eyes, and the segments of the tapeworms can occasionally be seen in the droppings.

TREATMENT: Withhold all food from eighteen to twenty-four hours, and to calves from two to eight months old give two teaspoonfuls of gasoline in a pint of milk. To yearlings, place one tablespoonful in a gelatin capsule and give with capsule gun. To cattle one year and over, place one ounce in capsule and give with capsule gun. Repeat this treatment two or three times during intervals of a week or two.

TEXAS FEVER

CAUSE: Due to a micro organism (Piropalasna Bigenium) which imbeds itself in the red blood corpuscles. This disease is transmitted or scattered by means of a tick which drops from the affected animal. The disease has various names, according to the locality in which it appears. Among them are: Spanish Fever, Red Water, Black Water, Red Murrian, Australian Cattle Tick Fever, etc.

SYMPTOMS: Loss of appetite. The animal ceases to ruminate, or does not chew the cud, and every sign of unthriftiness is displayed; a high temperature, and when the animal is standing the back is arched, but the animal, however, prefers to lie down most of the time and shows desire for solitude. The urine is very dark in color, hence the name "Red or Black Water." The disease is usually fatal, the animal dies within a few weeks.

TREATMENT: My advice is, when this disease once develops, or an animal shows any of the particular signs that I have mentioned, secure the services of a competent veterinarian, who will immunize by the use of serums, disinfectants, etc.

TICKS

Ticks are very difficult to kill, on account of their protected location, as ear ticks are not affected by dipping, and remedies strong enough for this purpose are liable to injure the animal, but these parasites may be expelled by pouring into the ear Carbolated Sweet or Cottonseed Oil with favorable results.

TUBERCULOSIS

CAUSE: The bacilli of Tuberculosis thrive in animals, especially those in a weakened condition, or when exposed to atmospheric changes, unwholesome food, dark and poorly ventilated stables. They gain entrance into the body through the lungs or the intestinal canal. They lodge in various portions of the lungs or intestines, and multiply very rapidly, causing irritations and formations, nodules, cysts or abscesses. They are the means of the bacillus entering the blood, which carries the infection to other parts of the body, as the spleen, liver, udder, womb, etc. Cows affected with generalized tuberculosis, that is to say, the infection is confined to not only a small portion of the lungs, but also to any of the above mentioned organs, etc., may give birth to a calf having general tuberculosis at birth, or shortly after, due to the cow's blood circulating through the body of the calf before birth.

SYMPTOMS: This disease may pass a casual observer unnoticed, although in some instances we notice a slight cough, unthriftiness, dullness. The coughing is best marked after taking a drink of water in the morning and then being exercised. Some animals keep up in good condition and look perfectly healthy while some get emaciated, have constipation, variable appetite, and sometimes growths or abscesses can be felt or seen in the udder or glands of the body and neck.

However, cattle showing any weakness, or the above symptoms, should be tested for tuberculosis by a competent veterinarian who has had the privileges of a veterinary education and experience in the administration of tuberculin.

TREATMENT: It is not advisable to treat tuberculosis. Thus far, medicine has failed to relieve the affected animal, or kill the bacillus of tuberculosis in a living animal. The infected animals should be disposed of on account of tubercular cows giving birth to tubercular calves, the milk being unfit for human consumption, unless it is thoroughly pasteurized. Infected cattle should be separated from healthy ones, as the disease spreads very rapidly. Drinking and feeding troughs are a means of spreading the infection, therefore, suspected cases of tuberculosis should be tested and if the animals react, they should be slaughtered, and if the disease is localized, passed for human consumption. The meat of animals suspected of having tuberculosis, or reacting from tuberculin test, should be well cooked.

TWISTED STOMACH WORM

CAUSE: Cattle become affected with this worm by grazing in pastures in which infested cattle have grazed and scattered their droppings. The worms in the stomach produce a multitude of eggs of microscopic size, which pass out of the body with the feces. In warm weather, these eggs hatch in a few hours; if the temperature remains about freezing point, they soon die. The eggs are also destroyed, by dryness, but, on the other hand, moisture, if the weather is warm, favors their development. The twisted worm measures one-half inch to one and one-half inches in length.

SYMPTOMS: General weakness, loss of flesh, anemia, dullness, capricious appetite, excessive thirst, paleness of the skin and mucous membranes of the mouth and eyes, and dropsical swelling, especially that of the lower jaw. Diarrhoea always accompanies this condition and if the feces is carefully examined the small worms may be seen wriggling about like little snakes, or when an animal dies; and the fourth stomach is opened, these worms can be seen in large quantities.

TREATMENT: Preventive measures are important, as damp, marshy soil favors the development of the embryos. High sloping ground is preferable for pasture. If low ground is used it should be properly drained; burning over the pasture will destroy most of the young worms on the grass and on the ground. Cattle should be supplied with water from flowing streams or wells and not stagnant ponds.

MEDICAL TREATMENT: Withhold all food for twenty-four hours; then administer Oil of Turpentine, placing it in an ounce capsule and give with capsule gun. Follow in six hours with a physic consisting of Aloin, two drams; ginger, two drams. Place in capsule and give with capsule gun. When this worm develops in calves, give as follows: One dram of Turpentine to a calf three months old, four drams to a calf six months old, six drams to a yearling. To cattle two years and over, give equivalent dose, or an ounce. The physic should be reduced in the same proportions as that of Turpentine.

VERMINOUS BRONCHITIS

(Lung Worms)

CAUSE: Due to worm or parasite called Strongylus Micrurus, a small thread-like worm two to four inches in length, found in the bronchial tubes, a portion of the lungs. The life history of this parasite is not known, but infection is apparently derived through the medium of pastures where infested cattle have grazed. Young cattle are more seriously affected than old animals, especially common in low marshy pastures.

SYMPTOMS: This form of bronchitis usually affects the entire herd; the animals become poor, unthrifty, hacking, coughing, especially at night, and sometimes animals actually cough up worms.

TREATMENT: Various treatments have been recommended for Verminous Bronchitis, or Lung Worm, as injecting Turpentine into the windpipe or fumigating animals by placing them in a closed shed or barn and burning sulphur, compelling the affected animals to inhale the fumes. This treatment perhaps is the safest and the most effective. A person should remain in the enclosed shed and when the fumes become so strong that there is danger of suffocation, open the doors and windows. This treatment should be repeated every week until coughing ceases.

WARBLES OR GRUBS

CAUSE: By the heel-fly or warble-fly. They deposit their eggs on the legs of cattle during the fall. The animal, licking the parts, takes the eggs into its mouth. These eggs gradually migrate into the gullet, where they hatch and burrow through the tissues, and in the early spring will be found in the region of the back in the form of small lumps under the skin.

SYMPTOMS: Warbles are frequently seen under the skin in the region of the back and over the loins, and are very tender to the touch. When they are fully developed they work their way through the skin, which usually occurs in the early part of the summer. Examine your cattle in the winter and spring for the presence of grubs. They can be easily found by running the hand over the loins, by abrupt swellings or bunches on the skin. Pressure on the swellings will perhaps cause the grubs to pop out.

TREATMENT: Remove the grubs by making a small incision with a clean, sharp knife in the center of the swelling. Then press them out and into each cavity from which the grub has been extracted, or squeezed out, should be injected a five per cent solution of Carbolized Sweet Oil to prevent any further development of flies or grubs. Cattle sprayed with fly repellants during the spring and summer are very seldom bothered with warbles or grubs. However, this is not practical in range cattle; dipping instead should be resorted to, and it is surprising what results will be derived from fly repellants in a year or two. They will practically exterminate the pest, and consequently the cattle are thrifty and look much better.

WARTS

CAUSE: Warts may appear on various parts of the body, and are due to an abnormal growth of cells growing upon the outer surface of healthy skin, or they may grow upon skin that is deprived of the proper blood supply.

TREATMENT: If the wart is located where there is hair surrounding it, cut away the hair, then wash the wart and surrounding parts with a five per cent solution of Carbolic Acid and clip the wart off with a sharp pair of scissors or knife. After the wart is removed, cauterize the cut surface with a hot iron. Caustic Potash or Silver Nitrate should be applied two or three times at the intervals of two or three days to insure the entire extermination of the wart. This same treatment applies to all classes of warts located in various places.

WHITES

(Leucorrhea)

CAUSE: Continual chronic inflammation of the womb, or due to irritations from a retained afterbirth. Injuries or wounds inflicted by hands or instruments in difficult calving, diseases of the ovaries, etc.

SYMPTOMS: A glarish, white discharge from the womb. When cow is lying down it flows more abundantly, soiling the tail, etc. The general health may not be much affected at first, but if the discharge continues and is putrid, the health fails, the milk shrinks, and there is a great loss of flesh. In some cases heat is more frequent or intense than natural, but the animal rarely conceives when served, and if she does, is likely to abort.

TREATMENT: Feed nitrogenous food. Wash the womb out with a solution consisting of five grains of Permanganate of Potash to one quart of water. This should be repeated once or twice a day. If the animal is constipated, give two drams of Aloin, three drams of Ginger. Place in gelatin capsule and give with capsule gun. Also place Potassium Iodide one dram, Hyposulphite of Soda one ounce in the drinking water two or three times a day. This not only diminishes the discharge, but has a good effect on the blood, particularly where there is more or less decomposition of the flesh.

WOLF IN THE TAIL

This condition is imaginary, although the muscles of the tail relax or soften, especially those of its extremity, due to ill health; consequently the condition of the cow should be treated, and not the tail.

TREATMENT: Remove the cause. Perhaps the animal has indigestion, or a cold, etc. Determine the malady by careful examination and treat the disease under its special heading.

It has been a custom among the so-called cow doctors to split the tail with a sharp knife, then fill the wound with salt and pepper and bandage with a cloth. This is a fallacy, and should not be tolerated.

DISEASES OF SWINE

Causes, Symptoms and Treatments

Location of Parts of Swine 1. Mouth 2. Nostrils 3. Face 4. Eyes 5. Ears 6. Jaws 7. Jowl 8. Neck 9. Shoulder 10. Fore flanks 11. Chest Floor 12. Pasterns 13. Dew Claw 14. Sheath 15. Belly 16. Side or ribs 17. Heart girth 19. Loin 20. Rump 21. Coupling 22. Rear flanks 23. Tail 24. Thighs 25. Hocks

CHAPTER III

HOG REGULATOR AND TONIC

Nux Vomica, one pound; Hardwood Charcoal, two pounds; Sulphur, two pounds; Common Salt, three pounds; Sulphide of Antimony, one and one-half pounds; Glauber Salts, two pounds; Bicarbonate of Soda, four pounds; Hyposulphite of Soda, four pounds; Nitrate of Potash, one pound; Quassia, one-half pound; Gentian Root, one pound; Iron Sulphate, one pound; pulverize and mix well.

To everyone hundred pounds of hog weight, give one tablespoonful in feed or swill once or twice daily. For hogs weighing two hundred pounds, the dose would be two tablespoonfuls; for a hog weighing fifty pounds, one-half tablespoonful.

Hogs, like other animals, require tonics, bowel regulators and worm expellers. For these purposes, I have prescribed under a number of the diseases of hogs, which I cover in this chapter, the above general tonic and regulator which I have used in my personal practice with marked success, especially serving the purpose of aiding hogs in their convalescence from debilitating diseases and in their recovery from a general run-down condition.

Aside from its general tonic and regulative effect, this prescription contains nerve tonics, intestinal antiseptics, laxatives, worm expellers, and aids digestion, etc.

If regularly given to hogs, and sanitary conditions are maintained, this tonic and regulator will largely fortify them against contagious diseases.

ABORTION

CAUSE: Sows may abort at any state of pregnancy by slipping, falling, receiving kicks, or by being caught while crawling through or under fences. Sows may also abort when allowed to crawl into quarters where there are other hogs. Contagious diseases, such as Cholera and Pleuropneumonia also produce abortion. There is also a contagious form of abortion in sows, but this is very uncommon, as the disease spreads very slowly.

SYMPTOMS: There is no warning given, as a rule; the sows expel their pigs before any signs of abortion are noticed.

In other cases the sows refuse to eat, become uneasy, shivering and trembling of the muscles, and straining or labor pains are noticed. As a rule, when a sow aborts, she will not prepare a bed, as she would normally.

TREATMENT: Preventive is the only safe and sure treatment, although when the first sign of abortion appears, and there are no signs of the membranes coming away, remove the sow to quiet, warm, clean quarters by herself, and if straining, give one dram of Chloral-Hydrate in her drinking water every two or three hours.

When a sow aborts, burn the pigs and afterbirth, and disinfect the pens with a Coal Tar disinfectant. Keep this up for several days, and do not breed until all discharges from the vagina have ceased flowing.

ADMINISTRATION OF MEDICINE TO HOGS

To administer medicine to hogs may seem easy, but, nevertheless, it is a difficult task. Never lay a hog on his back to drench him, as in so doing there is great danger of strangling. The proper method is to stand or set him on end, holding him up by the ears, and by the use of a bottle with a piece of hose drawn over its neck, give the medicine very slowly, so as not to allow a large quantity to accumulate in the mouth or throat at one time. There is always danger of some of the liquid escaping into the lungs and causing the hog to strangle, and thus it may produce pneumonia. However, this is the best method of giving hogs medicine by force.

Hogs will generally take medicine in their feed or drinking water, unless they are very sick, or the medicine is extremely disagreeable to the taste.

BAG INFLAMMATION

CAUSE: Injuries, obstructed teats, accumulation of milk in the sow's bag after the loss of part of or all of her litter. Difficult birth, slight wounds in the bag permit invasion of germs, which is frequently the common cause of bag inflammation.

SYMPTOMS: Heat, pain and swelling in one or more teats. The general body temperature is elevated one or two degrees above normal. The sow perhaps refuses her feed, although she will drink water in large quantities.

TREATMENT: Feed soft, sloppy food and vegetables. Give Epsom Salts, two to four ounces, in milk or feed. It is also well to milk the sow by hand, relieving her of the milk three or four times a day. This is very necessary. Camphorated Oil is very soothing, and I would recommend its use freely only over affected teats.

BLACK TOOTH

CAUSE: Black Tooth, so called in swine, is principally due to injuries to the teeth received by chewing hard matter, such as bone, etc., which causes them to decay.

SYMPTOMS: Toothache. Toothache in swine is similar to that exhibited by man, in showing loss of appetite, salivation, or slobbering, hanging the head mostly to the side which is affected, loss of fear of man, and offensive breath. If the hogs are fed on strongly acid food for any length of time, their teeth may become dark colored. As the teeth are not materially injured; so long as decayed tooth substance cannot be noticed, and while the appetite and chewing facilities of the hog do not appear to be diminished, no interference will be necessary.

It is customary with some people to examine the teeth of hogs, and if one tooth is found darker colored than the others, it is supposed to be the cause of the hog not doing well, if he is in a poor condition, and the tooth is hammered off flush with the jaw, leaving the broken roots, lacerated gums and nerves to increase the hog's suffering. If the hog recovers, it is often concluded that this was a case of Black Tooth.

My advice is, if you are determined to have the tooth out, extract it properly. Do not break it off. When your hogs are not thriving, give them the regulator and tonic prescribed on the first page of this chapter.

BLOOD POISONING

(Pyemia Septicemia)

CAUSE: Due to the toxic substance produced by germs that invade wounds, bruises, abscesses, or womb following farrowing, if lacerated.

SYMPTOMS: The seat of injury becomes swollen, pus may adhere to the hair, temperature elevated, appetite poor, hog moves about very slowly, becomes separated from the rest of the drove, lies around in some cool, quiet place, eventually becomes very weak and poor and dies, if good attention is not given.

TREATMENT: Separate from the other hogs and remove to a clean, comfortable place and wash the seat of injury with some good disinfectant, as a five per cent Carbolic Acid solution. In case of abscess, open it low so as to assure good drainage. Keep clean, cool water before your hogs at all times. Give mashes made from wheat bran and hot water, or any good, substantial food that is easily digested containing regulator and tonic prescribed on the first page of this chapter.

BRONCHITIS

CAUSE: Lung worms, poorly ventilated sleeping quarters, sleeping in straw stacks, in manure heaps, overheated, filthy pens, where the animals inhale irritating gases given off the bodies of other hogs, and from filth. Smoke and dust are very common producers of bronchitis.

SYMPTOMS: Breathing fast, appetite poor, slight rise in temperature and coughing. The hog is dull and stupid, refuses food, but drinks water frequently.

TREATMENT: Preventive; avoid the above named causes, but when hogs become affected, move them to clean, well ventilated quarters, avoiding dust and gases, disinfect bedding and floors with some good disinfectant, as Crude Carbolic Acid, sprayed. Also give large doses of the hog regulator and tonic, as prescribed on the first page of this chapter. Feed vegetables, or any easily digested food, and hot wheat bran mashes.

In case the disease is due to lung worms, confine the animals in a closed shed and permit them to inhale the steam from Turpentine and water for a few minutes, by placing water and Turpentine in a tin receptacle holding about two gallons, and inserting heated bricks or stones into the solution.

CASTRATION

This is generally understood by every stockraiser, yet there are some points many do not know. For instance, you should use in this operation an antiseptic solution, as Carbolic Acid or Bichloride of Mercury. Wash thoroughly with antiseptic yours hands and knife, also the seat of operation and make your incision as low as possible to permit the pus to drain out nicely. If this is not practiced, the pus will become absorbed into the blood, producing blood poison, which may produce death, or at the best will cause the hog to become stunted, whereas, if the operation is performed properly, the hog will thrive, regardless of the shock from the operation. I may add that it is much better to castrate pigs or hogs when their stomach and intestines are empty, and it is always good practice to feed laxative and easily digested foods sparingly after this operation.

CHOKING

CAUSE: Vegetables, such as potatoes, etc., roots, as carrots, turnips and sometimes pieces of bone or glass, lodge in the gullet. Paralysis of the muscular fibres of the gullet is a very common cause of choking in swine.

SYMPTOMS: The hog is unable to swallow, producing frothing at the mouth and, if the obstruction cannot be dislodged, death occurs in a very short time. Sometimes the obstruction in the gullet may be felt from the outside with the hand.

TREATMENT: The administration of small doses of Raw Linseed or Olive Oil, or Lard, will assist in dislodging the obstruction. Also careful manipulation of the gullet from the outside with the hand assists in either forcing it into the stomach or bringing it out through hog's mouth. If vomiting can be produced, it will dislodge the obstruction. If immediate results are not obtained from the above treatments, I would recommend butchering the hog for meat immediately.

COLD IN THE HEAD

(Nasal Catarrh)

CAUSE: Exposure to cold; a very common condition in cold, wet weather when hogs are allowed to sleep in manure heaps, straw stacks, or pile up together, when they become overheated and later chill. Nasal Catarrh may also be due to inhaling dust or irritating gases.

SYMPTOMS: The animal is stupid and feverish, coughing and sneezing frequently; appetite is poor, eyes watery and inflamed; a discharge of mucus from the nose will terminate in yellow pus and the nose, if examined, is found to be inflamed and ulcerated.

TREATMENT: The best and safest treatment is to provide clean sleeping quarters, avoid overcrowding in dusty, dirty sheds, especially during cold weather. Pigs affected with cold in the head should be fed on laxative food, such as boiled carrots, potatoes, apples, hot wheat bran mashes and steamed rolled oats.

MEDICAL TREATMENT: Confine the affected hogs to a shed, close windows and doors and any large cracks; then compel them to inhale steam from the following mixture: Turpentine, eight ounces; Pine Tar, one pint; Water, two gallons. Place in tin receptacle in center of shed and heat the above solution by adding hot bricks or stones to the mixture occasionally. Compel the hogs to inhale this steam for at least thirty minutes twice a day. Give Chlorate of Potash in twenty grain doses three times a day in feed or drinking water. This treatment is very successful if the inflammation has not extended to the lungs.

DIARRHOEA IN YOUNG PIGS

(Scours)

CAUSE: Decomposed foods, slops, etc., fed to the mothers, causing them to give toxic milk. Poorly ventilated, filthy, cold and damp pens, insufficient exercise, lack of sunlight, raising pigs by hand or with other sow.

SYMPTOMS: Frequent movement of the bowels, the passage being of a grayish-white color and the odor very disagreeable. At this stage of the disease, reliable remedies must be given or the pig will die very soon.

The discharge from the bowels becomes very thin, the tail and legs become soiled, loss of appetite, the pigs become weak and dull, hair rough and it is difficult for them to move about. In very young pigs, treatment is of little value.

TREATMENT: As Scours in pigs is a disease frequently caused by faulty food and insanitary surroundings, a preventive treatment is of great importance, and much better results are thus obtained than by the use of medical agents. Medical treatment consists in first cleaning away the irritant present in the bowels. For this purpose give one to two tablespoonfuls of Castor Oil. At the time of farrowing all sows should receive a light diet and be kept in clean, dry quarters. The pigs should be allowed pure air, sunshine and exercise. If the sow appears hot and feverish, give one to three ounces of Castor Oil in milk or swill. Avoid feeding decomposed, moldy food, or sour milk. To check the diarrhoea in pigs, use the following after the irritant is removed or cleaned out as above stated: Zinc Sulphocarbolates, thirty grains; Protan, two ounces; Pulv. Gentian Root, two ounces. Make into sixty capsules or powders and give one, three or four times a day. The sow should receive a dose about eight times the size of that of the pigs.

HOG CHOLERA

CAUSE: By the Bacillus Sius; contaminated food, stagnant water, filth, etc., all have a tendency to aid its progress. I have seen farms, although located in sections where Cholera was prevalent, not in the least troubled with the malady, perhaps due to careful feeding of clean foods, care in watering, cleanliness about the pens and sheds and disinfecting occasionally, but no doubt a better explanation is that those hogs received tonics, containing worm expellers, at least four times a year. Many a case of supposed Hog Cholera is due to worms irritating and producing inflammation of the intestines, followed by diarrhoea. A person not familiar with the disease calls this "hog cholera." In other cases, hogs which are fed swills from restaurants, hotels, etc., containing soap, washing powders, small particles of glass, etc., will die with symptoms leading a person to think they had Hog Cholera, but if a thorough investigation is made the true cause of death can easily be discovered.

SYMPTOMS: In true Hog Cholera, the temperature will be elevated two to four degrees above normal. There will be a loss of appetite, vomiting, diarrhoea, although there may be constipation when the hog is first affected. The hog wanders off by itself to some cool, quiet place and lies down. When it walks it will stagger and show great stiffness in its hind parts, due to soreness of the intestines. The hair will have a roughened appearance, the back arched, the eyes inflamed and discharging pus, red blotches will show themselves back of the ears, inside the legs and on the abdomen. At this stage the diarrhoea is watery, dark and tinged with blood, and very offensive in odor, breath is very fast and labored. The hog grows very weak and dies.

TREATMENT: Prevention must always be borne in mind. Do not feed filthy food. Always feed good, wholesome food, and give clean water to drink. Watch the condition of hog's bowels and regulate them by feeding. Burn manure and bedding and disinfect carefully. Do not permit your hogs to drink out of running streams of water, especially if Hog Cholera is in your neighborhood. When buying hogs, it is well to keep them off by themselves for two or three weeks, as they may be diseased. Do not permit neighbors, their stock or dogs on your premises when Hog Cholera is raging, as the infection of Hog Cholera can be spread very rapidly by matter from the affected hogs adhering to the shoes of man, to the feet of stock and dogs, etc.

I am positive that if this method were properly practiced by all hog raisers and feeders, Hog Cholera would be a very rare disease.

SERUM TREATMENT: This is successful in some cases, and in others unsuccessful. The latter perhaps is due to poor serums, or the disease being so far advanced in its progress that the hogs are beyond recovery. Serum treatment is very expensive and, as it requires a strictly septic operation of injecting the serum, the average hog raiser or grower is not qualified to administer the treatment properly. An additional and necessary expense is the services of a Veterinary Surgeon. Therefore, I strongly urge adoption of preventive measures as stated. Use some good disinfectant, such as Crude Carbolic Acid, which destroys the Bacillus of Hog Cholera. Also administer hog regulator and tonic as prescribed on first page of this chapter. This will expel worms, tone the system, regulate the bowels and fortify your hogs against Hog Cholera.

INDIGESTION

CAUSE: Worms are perhaps one of the most common causes. Unwholesome, irritating food or swill containing soap or washing powder have a tendency to derange the process of digestion.

SYMPTOMS: Abdominal pain, vomiting, back arched, breathing rapid and temperature elevated from two to three degrees. There may be diarrhoea or the animal may be constipated. Vomiting, as a rule, relieves acute attacks by expelling the irritant from the bowels. When it takes a chronic form, the hogs become stunted.

TREATMENT: Endeavor to find out the cause and remove it. If constipated, give Calomel, fifteen to twenty grains, or, if diarrhoea appears, give hog regulator and tonic as prescribed on first page of this chapter. Feed with hot wheat bran mashes. This will expel all worms and aid digestion.

JAUNDICE

(Yellows)

CAUSE: Liver flukes, intestinal worms, gall stones, lack of exercise, overfeeding, or a stoppage of the bile duct.

SYMPTOMS: The white portions of the eyes take on a yellow color, as do the membranes of the mouth, back arched, hair looks rough, vomiting, temperature elevated, constipation, although diarrhoea is sometimes noticed. The urine is passed frequently, and is of a dark amber color.

TREATMENT: This disease requires careful feeding and plenty of exercise. Give Calomel, ten to twenty grains, then follow with large doses of regulator and tonic as prescribed on first page of this chapter. It is important in this disease, especially if due to worms. Feed clean swill and vegetables. Give hogs all the pure water they will drink.

KIDNEY CONGESTION

CAUSE: Hogs are subject to various injuries about the kidneys, due to a large number of hogs piling up, exposure to cold, wet rains, etc.

SYMPTOMS: Small quantities of dark colored urine are passed frequently, appetite poor, no energy to move about. Hogs lie around a great deal; at times they may be paralyzed and drag their hind quarters.

TREATMENT: Apply cloths or blankets wrung out of hot water over the loin; also give Potassium Acetate in twenty grain doses four or five times a day in drinking water. Feed soft, sloppy food, containing regulator and tonic as prescribed on the first page of this chapter. It contains nerve stimulants, just what is required in paralysis.

KIDNEY WORM

CAUSE: Damp, filthy surroundings seem to favor the growth of embryos of this worm. They are taken into the digestive canal with the food and eventually pass to the region of the kidneys, where they find conditions favorable in which to multiply.

SYMPTOMS: May produce paralysis of the hind quarters, in which case the animal would not exhibit such marked tenderness on being pressed over the loins with the fingers as it would if the weakness of the hind quarters was due to a sprain or to rheumatism of the loins. Occasionally hogs may suffer from the presence of one or more worms in the kidneys; but the ailment is rarely fatal, becoming so only after a long time of suffering resulting in a degeneration of one or both kidneys. It is almost impossible to diagnose the presence of worms in the kidneys of hogs, except by chance through a microscopic examination of the urine. If worms are found in the kidneys of a hog that has died or been slaughtered for food it may then be reasonably supposed that other hogs of the same herd not acting normal are infected with worms of the same species.

TREATMENT: Teaspoonful doses of Turpentine in milk three times a week is the only treatment I could recommend. Preventive measures is the only practical method of treating a disease of this nature. Give your hogs pure water and food. Disinfect pens occasionally and keep them clean.

LICE ON HOGS

Dip, spray or scrub your hogs with some good Coal Tar disinfectant, but whatever remedy is used it should be applied more than once which, of course, causes considerable work where there is a large number of hogs infested, unless dipped, which is more quickly done. The reason for repeated applications being necessary is that although the lice which hogs pick up from the ground, bedding and rubbing places, may be killed by first application, it often does not affect the nits, which remain intact and hatch within a week or ten days. A new crop of Lice appears on the hog from this source. Remove all manure and bedding from pens and sheds and burn it. Disinfect floors and spray sides of shed, pens and rubbing places with disinfectants, one part to seventy-two parts of water, once a month and you will be handsomely repaid for your labor.

LUNG FEVER

(Inflammation of the Lungs)

CAUSE: Sudden changes, exposure to storms, piling up of hogs during cold nights, or sleeping in manure heaps, old straw stacks, etc.

SYMPTOMS: Pig or hog is taken with shivering spells, is stupid, his back is arched, loss of appetite, temperature elevated two to four degrees above normal, short hurried breathing, generally accompanied with cough, which is deep and hoarse. As a rule the hog is constipated.

TREATMENT: Place in good, clean, warm, well ventilated quarters, free from drafts. Keep water before them at all times, adding Saltpeter, one teaspoonful to every gallon of water. If constipated, do not give physics; give injections of soap and warm water; also administer about one-half teaspoonful of Pine Tar on the tongue with a wooden paddle. This adheres to the tongue and gradually dissolves and gives excellent results, as it is very soothing to the organs of breathing. During the convalescent stage, give hog regulator and tonic as prescribed on first page of this chapter.

LUNG WORMS

CAUSE: By threadlike worms varying in length from one-half to one and one-half inches and of a brownish-white color. They are found in the windpipe and tubes leading into the lungs. The adult worms in the lungs produce large quantities of eggs, which are coughed up with mucus and become scattered over premises where other hogs are permitted to walk. The hogs inhale the dust containing the eggs into their lungs, where the eggs find moisture sufficient for their development.

SYMPTOMS: Severe coughing spells. Large quantities of mucus will escape from the nose and mouth. The hog becomes stunted, although he may eat fairly well, but if not relieved, the worms collect in the Bronchi and produce sudden death due to suffocation. The worms may set up an inflammation of the lining membranes of the lungs, which is sometimes taken for Swine Plague, or Cholera. This disease is not uncommon, especially in old, filthy, poorly drained hog houses and pastures.

TREATMENT: Confine the affected hogs to a shed; close the windows and doors and any large cracks, then compel the hogs to inhale steam from the following mixture: Turpentine, eight ounces; Pine Tar, one pint; Water, two gallons. Place in tin receptacle in center of the shed and heat the above solution by adding hot bricks or stones to the mixture occasionally. Compel them to inhale this steam for at least thirty minutes twice a day. Feed wholesome food to which add hog tonic as prescribed on first page of this chapter. A strong, vigorous hog may have worms, but it retains its vitality so long as it is well fed.

MANGE

CAUSE: By the Sarcoptes Scabei. This parasite burrows under the outer surface of the skin.

SYMPTOMS: The parasite usually manifests itself on the skin under the armpits, thighs and inside of the fore legs. At first small red blotches or pimples appear, and these gradually spread as the parasites multiply and burrow under the skin.

TREATMENT: There is no other way of curing this disease, or of preventing it, than by killing the parasites and their eggs; not only on the pigs themselves, but also on the sides of the pens, sheds, rubbing-posts, or anything that an affected hog rubs against.

When treating this disease, the real aim must be to kill the parasite by the prompt and continuous use of external remedies, such as washing or dipping, which is better done with some good disinfectant, one part to seventy parts water. Repeat this every ten days until cured. Two dippings are generally sufficient. It is well to feed cooling foods, such as clean slops and vegetables, containing regulator and tonic as prescribed on first page of this chapter.

NAVEL RUPTURE

(Navel or Umbilical)

CAUSE: Injuries. Pigs crowding through narrow doorways or openings in fences, small pigs sleeping with large pigs, and allowed to pile up, or being thrown about feed troughs when feeding. Weakness and constipation also predisposes them to Navel or Umbilical Rupture.

SYMPTOMS: A soft, puffy swelling about the navel or umbilicus, varying in size from a hazelnut to that of an ostrich egg. When a pig is placed on its back the intestines will gravitate into the abdominal cavity, providing the intestines have not adhered to the walls of the rupture.

TREATMENT: This is more difficult than the Scrotal or Inguinal Rupture operation, as often times the intestines will adhere to the inner surface of the rupture and, unless the operation is carefully performed, there is great danger. Great care must be exercised in preparing the pig by fasting it for twenty-four hours. After this is accomplished, prepare an antiseptic solution, Carbolic Acid, five per cent, or Bichloride of Mercury, one in one-thousandths; also have a needle and absorbent silk or cat-gut ready. Place the pig on its back, with its head downward. Now, wash the seat of operation with either antiseptic solution. Then make an incision through the skin carefully; as stated before, intestines sometimes adhere to the inner surface of the rupture. If such is the case, wash the hands in the antiseptic solution and with the fingers carefully break the adhesions or separate the intestines from their adhesions. After this is accomplished, sew the inner lining of the abdominal cavity with absorbent silk or cat-gut. Then sew the outer skin with cotton or linen cord and your operation is complete. Feed the hog sparingly for a few days following the operation on easily digested, laxative foods.

NETTLE RASH

(Urticaria)

CAUSE: Irritations of the skin produced by sprinkling hogs with irritating solutions and powders, or from irritating dips when treating for lice, etc.

Feeding highly nitrogenous food predisposes hogs to this disease; also filth, poorly drained sheds and pens; is especially common in young pigs. Nettle Rash is not contagious, but what produces it in one hog may produce it in several at the same time.

SYMPTOMS: Red, swollen blotches appear on the skin very suddenly, especially about the ears and the inside of the thighs, perhaps due to the skin being thin and deprived of hair. The hog rubs it on account of the intense itching, and he will not thrive when in this condition. In most cases there is a fluid oozing from the blotches, causing dirt and filth to adhere to the hair. However, if the disease is properly treated, a recovery is sure to follow in about two weeks.

TREATMENT: Prevention against this disease is most important, and it consists in keeping shoats and pigs in clean, well ventilated sheds and pens. Do not sprinkle them with irritating solutions or powders, or irritating dips, but when the disease once shows itself give each pig or hog affected a dose of Epsom Salts, one ounce to every twenty-five pounds of hog weight, in feed, swill or drinking water. If the weather is hot, keep them in a clean, cool place, also purify their blood by feeding regulator and tonic as prescribed on first page of this chapter.

Apply some good Coal Tar disinfectant, one part to one hundred parts of water. This is non-irritating, and will destroy hog lice, and will heal the pustules of nettle rash. Apply twice ten days apart. It also must be borne in mind that pens and sleeping quarters must be disinfected; the old bedding and manure burned and replaced with good, clean straw or hay. Feed easily digested food, slops, etc.

PARALYSIS OF THE HIND QUARTERS

CAUSE: There are a great many things that may produce paralysis of the hind quarters. For instance, shipping hogs in crates; fractions of thigh bones; Rickets, due to feeding food that is deficient in mineral matter; hogs piling up; kicks or injuries to the back; frequently seen in sows nursing a litter of pigs and in a run-down condition. Constipation and indigestion also produce paralysis of the hind quarters. Some think it is caused by worms in the kidneys; this is not always the case. It is true that the presence of a parasite around the kidneys may cause irritation of the nerves of the spinal column and result in paralysis. Yet, it is more often the result of weakness and loss of nervous power of the hind parts.

SYMPTOMS: Regardless of the cause, the symptoms in either case, for they cannot be distinguished, are weakness of the back, wriggling of the hind parts, and finally the hogs sit down on their haunches. After some effort, they get up and run in a straight line quite fast, but swing to one side for a while and then go over to the other side, and finally get down so that they cannot rise, but drag themselves about. The appetite is good until a day or two before they die.

TREATMENT: Place the hog in clean, comfortable quarters, with plenty of fresh water to drink. Give sour milk, fruit or vegetables, containing regulator and tonic as prescribed on first page of this chapter. It contains nerve stimulants and blood purifiers. If the hog is constipated, add two to four ounces of Epsom Salts to its feed. Treatment of all such cases requires perseverance, recovery being slow and not always certain.

PILES

(Prolapse of the Anus)

CAUSE: Although the pig may look well, he has a weakness of the circular fibres of the intestines, due to irritating foods that either constipate or produce diarrhoea.

SYMPTOMS: Very plain. A protrusion of the rectum all the way from two to four inches. The pig irritates the protrusion by rubbing it against the sides of pens, etc.; it cracks, bleeds and in warm weather will become fly-blown and maggots accumulate in large quantities.

TREATMENT: In the first stages of this disease, wash the protruded parts with an antiseptic solution of Carbolic Acid, one teaspoonful to a pint of water. Give rectal injections of Soap and Warm Water or Sweet Oil, give about two ounces of Castor Oil internally and feed soft, sloppy food. In chronic cases of long standing, remove the exposed portion of the intestine after washing nicely with the antiseptic solution. Remove the protrusion with a sharp knife and stitch the cut end of intestine edges to the anus. Feed easily digested food, such as wheat bran, mixed with flaxseed meal on which boiling hot water has been poured, cooling before feeding. Also give regulator and tonic as prescribed on first page of this chapter.

PIN WORMS

CAUSE: Hogs consume the eggs that encapsule well matured embryonic worms with their food or drinking water. These worms multiply very rapidly in the small intestines and are from one-half to one inch in length.

SYMPTOMS: No signs are noticed unless the worms are very abundant, as they are small and difficult to see with the naked eye. The principal point of attack is in the back part of the small intestines, where considerable inflammation is set up, especially when there are other worms, such as the Roundworm, present.

TREATMENT: Is of little value, as the worms in the intestines are very difficult to get at, but as their presence causes very little disturbance, it is hardly worth while treating; however, preventive measures should be applied by disinfecting, burning manure and bedding.

The following has proven a very effective treatment for Pinworms: Powdered Quassia, one pound; Sulphur, two pounds; Glauber Salts, one pound; Powdered Tobacco, one-half pound; Sulphide of Antimony, one pound; Hyposulphite of Soda, two pounds; Beechwood Charcoal, one pound; Common Salt, two pounds.

The above must be well powdered and thoroughly mixed. Give one heaping teaspoonful to everyone hundred pounds of hog weight. To small pigs, give doses in proportion to weight. Place it in their feed or slop twice a day. In addition to being a vermifuge, it is an alterative and tonic that should be given pigs and hogs which do not thrive properly. Best results are obtained in treatment of Pinworm when the principal food consists of vegetables, mashes and slops.

PLEURISY

CAUSE: Exposure to cold, damp, chilly weather, especially to drafts, or by a large number of hogs being allowed to pile up during cold nights, etc.

SYMPTOMS: Chilling, temperature elevated two or three degrees above normal; breathing fast. The hog will show great pain when pressed over the lungs by flinching, squealing or grunting; coughing suppressed, ribs rigid; breathing mostly with the muscles of the flanks; appetite poor and eventually there will be fluids accumulate in the lung cavities. At this stage, the breathing is labored and difficult. If the ear is pressed over the lungs, the fluids can be heard, and in the first stage the sound will be similar to that of rubbing hair between the finger and thumb.

TREATMENT: Remove the cause. The treatment is satisfactory if applied in due time. Place in clean, comfortable shed, seeing that it is well ventilated, omit drafts; apply equal parts of Aqua Ammonia Fort., Turpentine and Sweet Oil over the lungs and give two or four ounces of Castor Oil in milk. Feed easily digested food, such as hot wheat bran mashes, containing hog regulator and tonic as prescribed on first page of this chapter. It is also well to feed vegetables.

RHEUMATISM

CAUSE: Exposure, as in cold, damp houses. Overfeeding also has a tendency to cause swellings of the joints and muscles.

SYMPTOMS: Lameness of one or more limbs, swelling of the joints about the legs and feet. The hog does not care to move, refusing its feed in most cases; temperature slightly elevated; breathing quick and short; he will drink water frequently if offered.

TREATMENT: I am of opinion that Rheumatism in hogs would be a very rare disease if they were properly provided with clean, dry quarters, with a liberal quantity of bedding. Do not allow hogs to pile up, as it is very injurious to them.

MEDICAL TREATMENT: Consists of feeding sloppy food to which add one-half dram of Sodium Salicylate two or three times a day in their feed. Vegetables and green grass are very beneficial in this disease, as they have a cooling effect on the blood. The hog tonic and regulator recommended on first page of this chapter is very beneficial when given with food of a sloppy nature.

RICKETS

CAUSE: Food deficient in mineral matter or lime; filth, lack of exercise, and crowded quarters, all tend to produce a softening of the bones and swelling of the joints.

SYMPTOMS: The pigs affected generally appear in good condition and seem to be doing well, but suddenly they become paralyzed in the hind quarters, owing to the weakened condition of the bones, which sometimes fracture without receiving injury or any additional weight to that of the pig itself. The bones of the snout, back, limbs and feet bend and become deformed. The pigs grow weak, poor and stunted and perhaps the best treatment is to destroy them.

PREVENTIVE TREATMENT: Careful feeding of good, wholesome food. This disease is very seldom seen where hogs are frequently fed corn.

MEDICAL TREATMENT: When the first signs of Rickets appear, feed regulator and tonic as prescribed on first page of this chapter. It contains the mineral matter needed by the hog.

ROUND WORMS

CAUSE: Is undoubtedly due to filth or hogs eating food or drinking water contaminated with well developed eggs or embryos of roundworms, thus taking them into their digestive canal, where they multiply rapidly and set up considerable irritation. This worm varies in length from three to thirteen inches, and is of a reddish-brown color.

SYMPTOMS: The Roundworm is generally passed with the feces, and can be readily seen with the naked eye. A hog infested with a large number of these worms is generally restless, appetite varied. When these worms develop in large numbers, they obstruct the intestines. In other cases they irritate and inflame the intestines causing inflammation and diarrhoea, and death may be due to either obstruction or inflammation of the bowels.

TREATMENT: Treatment is very satisfactory. Withhold all food from eighteen to twenty-four hours. Then place in one pint of finely ground feed, Calomel and Santonin, each five grains to every one hundred pounds of hog weight. For instance, if the hog affected with round worms weighs two hundred pounds, double the dose by giving ten grains of each of the above, but if the hog only weighs fifty pounds, give one-half the dose mentioned, or two and one-half grains of each. This treatment should be repeated in a week or ten days to assure the expulsion of worms that might have survived the first dose. Feed sparingly on laxative food, as bran mashes and vegetables, for a few days following each treatment.

RUPTURE

(Scrotal or Inguinal)

DEFINITION: In the male the intestines pass through the wide Inguinal Canal, through which the cord of the testicle passes. It is not difficult to recognize this form of rupture, as the scrotum that normally retains only the testicles is usually enlarged by the bowels entering it. Sometimes the scrotum almost reaches the ground, and in this case, both sides of the scrotum, or the sack which contains the testicles, also contains intestines. If the pig is held up by the hind parts, the intestines will gravitate back into the abdominal cavity, but as soon as a pig lies down or stands they again return into the scrotum. The testicles can be located at the bottom of the enlargement.

CAUSE: Hereditary tendencies predisposes them to rupture; pigs having large Inguinal Canals through which the testicle passes; by pigs being crowded, injured, squeezed at troughs, or passing through narrow doorways. Weakness and severe straining from constipation also produce rupture.

SYMPTOMS: An enlargement of the sack containing the testicles. Sometimes there may be a strangulation of the intestines where they fold or twist. They become inflamed and produce death. The pig dies in great pain, but fortunately, strangulated ruptures in pigs are very rare, as the scrotum and canal which the intestines occupy relax and become very roomy.

TREATMENT: Operation is the only method of relieving or curing Inguinal or Scrotal Rupture. My advice is to operate as soon as possible. When the pigs are small, there is less danger. The pig to be operated on should be fasted for at least twenty-four hours, as it is easier on both the operator and pig when the intestines are empty, or nearly so.

The operation which I have found to be very successful is as follows: Have an assistant hold the pig up by its hind legs. Prepare an antiseptic solution of Carbolic Acid five per cent, or Bichloride of Mercury, one in one-thousandths, in a pan. Have a needle threaded with a medium sized absorbent silk or cat-gut suture. Prepare a clean, sharp knife; wash the seat of operation with either antiseptic solution. Now, proceed to locate the testicle by having the hind parts elevated. The intestines must be pressed back into the abdominal cavity. The testicle will remain in the sack or scrotum; now grasp the testicle between the fingers and make the incision through the scrotum and to the lower portion. It may be necessary to insert two fingers to withdraw the testicle. When the testicle is located, withdraw it. Before cutting it off it is well to run a needle containing a thread through the last covering of the testicle so as to prevent the membrane from returning. After this is securely done, remove the testicle and sew the inner membranes that envelop the rupture and testicle with what is called a "tobacco pouch suture." Draw it together firmly and tie and cut off suture about one-half inch from the knot. Your operation is now complete. Do not sew the outer incision in the scrotum, as it would have a tendency to accumulate dirt and hold pus. It should have a free drainage. Wash with one of the above mentioned antiseptics twice daily until thoroughly healed. Also feed laxative foods that are easily digested.

SORE FEET

CAUSE: Filth; especially common in large hogs when confined to hard floors or driven over rough, hard roads, or continually kept in filthy pens. The tissues of the feet become softened, especially those between the claws. Irritation is set up by germs entering the abrasions.

SYMPTOMS: The hogs will be noticed going very lame and if closely examined the above named conditions will be found.

TREATMENT: Remove the hogs to clean, dry pens containing plenty of clean bedding, and wash the affected parts with some good disinfectant, as five per cent solution of Carbolic Acid. Repeat this treatment at least once a day. In case the feet are badly inflamed, I would advise the application of hot Flaxseed Meal poultices to the feet. Feed easily digested food, as it aids materially in the treatment of infectious wounds.

SORE MOUTH

CAUSE: Decomposed foods. Also slops or stagnant water, washing powders, broken glassware, etc., from the tables, fed in slops, barley or wheat beards, etc.

SYMPTOMS: Difficulty in eating, or refusal to eat at all. Stringy secretions of saliva continually oozing from the mouth. The mouth gives off very offensive odor.

TREATMENT: In this form of sore mouth, remove the cause. Feed soft, wholesome food, such as wheat bran mashes and vegetables. In cases where it is due to the lodging of beards of wheat or barley, gag the hog's mouth with a piece of wood and remove the beards with forceps. Keep clean, cool water before them at all times and avoid feeding dry, hard food.

SOWS EATING THEIR YOUNG

CAUSE: Insufficient lime or mineral matter fed prior to farrowing; constipation is also a fruitful cause.

PREVENTION: Careful feeding for a few days prior to farrowing of slops, free from soap or washing powders; cool food, such as wheat bran mashes, with hog tonic and regulator as prescribed on the first page of this chapter. This is loosening to the bowels and also contains mineral matter and blood purifiers which are very valuable in the above mentioned condition.

SUN OR HEAT STROKE

CAUSE: Hogs that are very fat, and driven, hauled or shipped to market when the weather is warm, are frequently stricken with heat or sun-stroke. Sometimes when hogs are overcrowded and not protected from the rays of the sun, or from heat, they may become victims of heat or sunstroke.

SYMPTOMS: First they stagger when walking, then they become very weak and temperature elevates three or four degrees higher than normal. Prostration or extreme depression, or sometimes involuntary spasms or contractions of muscles occur.

TREATMENT: Prevention. Do not drive, haul or ship during the hottest part of the day, hogs that are not accustomed to exercise or extreme heat. Do not crowd hogs in small pens or sheds during the hot months, as their bodies give off considerable heat in addition to that of the sun. See that they are protected from the sun. When hauling or shipping hogs, wet them occasionally with water. It prevents heat stroke. In case a hog is suffering from heat or sun-stroke, place it in a cool, shady place and apply ice or cold water to the head only. Also give Saltpeter in teaspoonful doses every six hours diluted in one ounce of water. Also give Alcohol, one teaspoonful, every three hours in one ounce of water. Good recovery is often obtained from the above treatment.

THORN-HEADED WORMS

CAUSE: A white grub that is found in old manure heaps, straw stacks and hog lots carries eggs containing embryos of the Thorn-headed Worm. The white grub is eaten by the hog. The larvae of the Thorn-headed Worm is liberated by the process of digestion and becomes a parasite in the intestines of the hogs, where it develops into a fully matured worm. Large numbers of hogs quickly become infested with this parasite, as they multiply very rapidly. These worms vary from two to twelve inches in length, and have a whitish color.

SYMPTOMS: As a general rule, a worm can be seen in the feces. Other signs are that the hog loses flesh, appetite irregular, constipation, and then again there may be diarrhoea, especially where there are large numbers of worms present.

TREATMENT: First of all, burn all manure or decomposed vegetation that the hogs are liable to come in contact with. Withhold all food from eighteen to twenty-four hours and give one teaspoonful of Oil of Turpentine to everyone hundred pounds of hog weight, or if the hog weighs less than one hundred pounds, doses should be given in proportion. Follow this treatment for three or four consecutive days. Turpentine is easily given to hogs, as they will drink it in milk when well mixed. Perhaps it is advisable, where a large number of hogs are affected, to divide them into pens of five or ten hogs, as they are thus less likely to get an overdose. Feed laxative food. Clean and disinfect troughs and feeding floors. Also give prescription on first page of this chapter.

THUMPS

CAUSE: Disorders of the digestive system from overloading the stomach and causing irritation of the nerves leading to the diaphragm, which is the membrane that separates the lungs and heart from the intestines, stomach, liver and spleen. It is a spasm of this membrane that causes a hog or pig to have "Thumps." Insufficient exercise; a large number of pigs may become affected at the same time when closely confined.

SYMPTOMS: Jerking of the flanks; the pig or hog becomes very weak and stunted in a very short time.

TREATMENT: Remove the cause. In pigs, when first affected, careful feeding and exercise will generally effect a cure. In some cases, where the pigs are very small, it is well to take them away from the mother, permitting them to nurse very little. Give them Castor Oil in teaspoonful doses, and compel them to exercise. It may be necessary to give them Chloral Hydrate ten to fifteen grains two or three times a day diluted in a teaspoonful of water. Where the pigs will not eat mashes or drink milk, give them medicine by force with a teaspoon.

AFTER TREATMENT: Give hog regulator and tonic as prescribed on first page of this chapter.

WHIP WORM

This worm is very uncommon, but occasionally is found in the large intestines.

CAUSE: The eggs become imbedded in the manure, bedding, etc., and then mix with the feed and drinking water and are taken into the digestive canal where they develop into matured worms. This worm is from one to three inches in length, the hind extremity of which is very thin, hence the name, "Whipworm."

SYMPTOMS: They produce very little disturbance, even though present in large quantities, except when other worms assist in their irritating the lining membranes of the large intestines.

MEDICAL TREATMENT: Withhold all food from eighteen to twenty-four hours, then give one teaspoonful of Gasolene thoroughly mixed with milk, to everyone hundred pounds of hog weight. Small hogs, reduce the dose in proportion to their weight. It is advisable to follow this dose for two or three consecutive days. Feed food that is easily digested, and see that they have fresh water to drink.

DISEASES OF SHEEP AND GOATS

Causes, Symptoms and Treatments

1. Mouth 2. Nostrils 3. Eyes 4. Forehead 5. Poll 6. Ears 7. Neck or Scrag 8. Throat or Throttle 9. Brisket or Breast 10. Shoulder vein 11. Shoulder 12. Legs 13. Fore flank 14. Heart girth 15. Crops 16. Back 17. Loin 18. Rump 19. Coupling 20. Ribs 21. Belly 22. Sheath 23. Scrotum 24. Rear flanks 25. Leg of Mutton 26. Twist 27. Tail or Dock 28. Rump

CHAPTER IV

ABORTION

CAUSE: Is usually produced by injuries, or by the ewes being poisoned from eating poisonous foods, plants, etc. It has never occurred in infectious form in this country, although sometimes an outbreak is thought infectious on account of several ewes aborting about the same time, but all such outbreaks have been traced to some irritating poison which they had taken with their food or drinking water.

PREVENTIVE TREATMENT: Remove the aborted lambs or kids and afterbirth from the yards, and also withdraw the ewe or nanny and place her in comfortable quarters. She requires care and extra nursing, or she will become very poor and lose a large portion of her fleece.

MEDICAL TREATMENT: If due to poisonous plants, etc., when the first symptoms of Abortion or poisoning are noticed, give six to ten ounces of Castor Oil. Warm the oil so it will run freely. Set the sheep or goat upon its haunches and pour very slowly. Great care must be exercised so as not to let any of the oil enter the lungs, as it may produce fatal pneumonia. Feed food that is easily digested and supply them with pure water to drink. When the general condition is weak or run down, so to speak, the following tonic is recommended: Pulv. Gentian Root, one ounce; Pulv. Nux Vomica, one ounce; Pulv. Potassium Nitrate, one ounce; Hyposulphite of Soda, three ounces; Protan, three ounces. Mix and make into twenty-four powders. Give one powder two or three times daily well back on the tongue.

REMEMBER all tonics are bitter, therefore beware of any so-called tonics that the animals eat readily as these possess no real tonic values.

BLACK SCOURS

(Verminous Gastritis--Strongylosis)

CAUSE: Due to a worm (Strongylus Contortus) measuring one-fourth to one inch in length, inhabiting the intestines and the fourth stomach of sheep and goats. This disease is frequently seen in low, marshy pastures, where animals infested with the worm pass the ova or egg with the feces, the eggs developing into an embryotic worm which is again taken with the food or water by non-infected animals, whereby this disease again attacks the intestines and fully matured worms develop.

SYMPTOMS: Naturally, the symptoms vary according to the violence of the attack. In well developed cases, the animal strains to defecate, and passes shreds of intestinal mucous along with blood-stained feces. Finally a severe dysentery takes place, the animal becomes correspondingly weak, and death takes place in two or three days. Some cases become chronic, in which death does not take place for a month or more. However, the latter is uncommon. Other signs are staggering gait, trembling, eyes fixed, showing wild expression, neck turned to one side. Then the animal appears as if in pain, and looks around at the flank frequently. There is a chopping of the jaws, and a very free flow of stringy saliva dropping from the mouth. When an animal dies from the symptoms just described, it should be cut open and carefully examined for this particular parasite, which can be easily seen with the naked eye.

TREATMENT: Very successfully treated when the first symptoms appear by administering one ounce of Gasolene with a pint of Milk. To lambs or kids give half the dose. Every precaution should be taken so as to prevent the drench from entering the lungs. Perhaps the best method is to set the animal on its haunches and pour the liquid slowly and carefully; if they cough, let them down. Any drench entering the lungs produces fatal pneumonia. Feed good nourishing food, and supply them with fresh water to drink.

CATARRH

(Cold in the Head)

CAUSE: Atmospheric changes, sudden exposure to cold, wet weather after being accustomed to warm, comfortable surroundings, inhaling dust, smoke and gases or, in fact, anything that will produce an irritation to the membranes lining the nose; commonly seen in the spring and fall.

SYMPTOMS: Chilling, elevation of temperature, nose dry, breathing hurried, sneezing, coughing, dullness, appetite varied. In the first stages of the malady, the nostrils are considerably inflamed, but in the course of a few days the temperature subsides and a yellowish-white discharge flows from the nose continuously.

TREATMENT: Keep the affected animals dry, omit drafts, feed good, wholesome food, and provide bedding for them to lie upon. In the first stages of this malady, it is advisable to confine the animals in a barn, closing the windows and doors and compelling them to inhale steam from boiling hot water and Pine Tar. The best method to accomplish this is by placing a tub about half full of water in the center of the barn and add about one gallon of Pine Tar. Then heat bricks or stones and place them into the tub. In this way a large number can be treated at one time. The sheep should be compelled to inhale this steam for thirty to forty minutes twice a day. In addition to the above, the following is very beneficial: Chlorate of Potash, one ounce; Nitrate of Potassi, two ounces. Make into sixteen powders and give one powder to each sheep in its drinking water two or three times daily. Feed hot bran mashes and vegetables if possible.

DIARRHOEA

(Dysentery)

CAUSE: Diarrhoea, or Dysentery, is a sign of some irritation of the intestines resulting in increased secretions, or increased muscular contraction, or both. The irritation is sometimes the result of chilling from exposure, improper feeding, as contaminated or frozen foods, irritating foods, drinking cold or stagnant water, indigestion, organic diseases of the intestines, or parasitic diseases. (See Strongylosis.)

SYMPTOMS: Movements from the bowels are frequent, at first consisting of thin fecal matter, but as this malady progresses it becomes watery and offensive in smell, and streaked with blood. At first the animal shows no constitutional disturbances, but eventually it becomes weak and shows signs of abdominal pain by looking around to the flank, throwing the feet together, lying down, or moving restlessly. Sometimes this disease is accompanied by fever, great depression, loss of strength, rapid loss of flesh; terminating in death.

TREATMENT: Determine the cause and remove it if possible. When the disease is due to irritating properties of food which have been fed the animal, it is well to give a physic of Castor Oil in two to six ounce doses, according to the size of the animal. When there is debility, want of appetite, and temperature normal, but continuous water discharge from the bowels, give Protan, two ounces; Gum Catechu, one ounce; Pulv. Ginger, one ounce; Zinc Sulphocarbolates, eight grains. Make into sixteen powders and give one powder on the tongue every three or four hours, according to the severity of the attack. Feed food that is easily digested, as wheat bran mashes, steamed rolled oats, etc. See that the drinking water is fresh and clean.

FOOT ROT

(Foul in the Foot)

CAUSE: Foot Rot is produced by inflammation of the soft structures of the foot between the claws or toes. It may be due to an overgrowth and inward pressure, etc., or from filth accumulating and hardening between the claws, producing inflammation and softening or ulceration of the skin in the interdigital space (between the claws). Under some conditions several sheep or goats in the same drove become affected at the same time, leading many to think that the disease is contagious. When Foot Rot appears in a very short time, among sheep or goats, this condition can almost always be traced to filth, irritation, etc.

SYMPTOMS: The animal is observed to limp when walking. On careful examination of the foot we find it hot, swollen above the claws and in the soft parts between them, frequently spreading the claws apart to a considerable extent, or the inflammation may have advanced to softening and sloughing of the soft structure between the claws. If this condition is neglected at this stage, deep abscesses form and the pus burrows under the horny wall, and the joints within the hoof become inflamed and destroyed, in which case the treatment is difficult and recovery will be very arduous.

TREATMENT: In the early stages of the disease, before the pus burrows beneath the horny structures of the foot, any foreign substances impacted between the claws should be removed. Then place a trough about one foot wide, six to eight inches high, and twelve to sixteen feet long, and fill with water and Coal Tar Dip, diluted in proportions of one part dip to fifty parts of water. Build a fence on each side of the trough, just wide enough for one sheep to pass through, and compel every sheep to walk through the solution slowly.

This treatment should be repeated once or twice a week until the lameness has disappeared. In cases where deep sloughing has taken place under the horny structures, saturate a piece of oakum or cotton in the following liniment: Oil of Origanum, Oil of Pisis, Oil of Turpentine, each four ounces. Place it between the claws and hold it there by means of a bandage. Repeat this application every other day. The animals that do not show signs of improvement under this treatment in a few days invariably have the joints of the foot affected and should not be driven.

FORAGE POISONING

CAUSE: This condition is produced by animals eating various foliage (Grass or Shrubbery) at a time when the peculiar poisonous principles are developed in it, as appears to happen in certain seasons. The disease is liable to affect a large proportion of animals which are under the same grazing conditions.

SYMPTOMS: Generally takes two or three days to develop. The animal gradually becomes more or less unconscious and paralyzed, staggers when forced to walk, and it may have great difficulty in keeping on its feet, it is extremely averse to going down, and leans for support against any convenient object. It breathes in a snorting manner. The mucous membranes are tinged with yellow, and the bowels constipated. In other cases severe diarrhoea follows, and the animal becomes very weak and dies in convulsions or spasms. Recovery may be expected in cases that are not marked by severe symptoms.

TREATMENT: Endeavor to find out the true cause and remove it if possible. Change range or pasture for a short time; this has successfully eradicated this malady. The animal showing the above symptoms should receive four to eight ounces of Castor Oil regardless of whether there is diarrhoea or constipation. In either case the irritation will be relieved by its laxative effect. In cases where diarrhoea becomes chronic, after administering the Castor Oil, the following will be found very efficient in its control: Protan, three ounces; Ginger, one ounce; Gum Catechu, two ounces. Make into sixteen powders and place one powder well back on the tongue every four or six hours. Feed clean, wholesome food and supply clean, fresh water to drink. Provide shelter for the animal if the weather is hot.

GARGET

(Congestion and Inflammation of the Udder)

CAUSE: As a rule, in Garget or Congestion of the Udder in heavy milking ewes, just before and after lambing, the glands of the udder enlarge, become hot, tense and tender and a slight pasty swelling extends forward from the glands on the lower surface of the abdomen. This physiological condition is looked upon as a matter of course and disposed of in two or three days when the secretions of milk have been fully established. General breaking up of the udder may be greatly hastened by the sucking of a hungry lamb and the kneading it gives the udder with its nose is beneficial. The above mentioned congestion or Garget may emerge into active inflammation resulting from continued exposure to cold weather, standing in cold drafts or injury to the udder from stone, clubs, feet of other animals, overfeeding or rich food, like cotton seed or soy bean, sore teats or a ewe losing her lamb in the period of full milking; serious disturbances of the animal's health is liable to fall upon the udder.

SYMPTOMS: The symptoms and mode of attack vary in different cases. Following exposure to cold drafts or cold, wet weather, there is usually severe chilling with cold ears and limbs and general dryness and brittleness of the wool. This is followed by a flush of heat, the ears and limbs become unnaturally warm and the glands swell up and become firm and solid in one or both sides of the udder. The muzzle is hot and dry, temperature elevated two or three degrees above normal, pulse firm and quick, excited breathing, appetite and rumination suspended, bowels constipated, urine scanty and the yield of milk may be entirely suppressed in the affected side.

TREATMENT: Determine the cause and remove it if possible. Move the affected animal to comfortable quarters, supply liberal quantifies of bedding for the animal to lie upon. Give two to six ounces of Glauber Salts dissolved in a pint of hot water. Permit it to cool. Place the ewe on her haunches and drench carefully. Feed laxative foods as hot bran mashes, steamed rolled oats and vegetables, supplying the animal with pure water to drink, to which add two drams of Hyposulphite of Soda, two or three times a day. In some cases it is advisable to apply Camphorated Ointment to the udder once or twice a day.

GID

(Sturdy)

CAUSE: Gid is produced by a bladder worm, a larva or an egg of the tapeworm infesting the intestines of dogs, wolves and coyotes. The eggs of these tapeworms are scattered over the range or pastures in the droppings of infested dogs, wolves or coyotes, and these when swallowed in the food or water by the sheep, hatch out and the embryos migrate to the brain, spinal cord, etc., where they develop into cysts, bladder worms or water bags, etc. When the organs of sheep, thus infested, are eaten by dogs, wolves or coyotes, the cyst worms are also likely to be swallowed and then develop into mature tapeworms.

SYMPTOMS: In case a large number of embryos become lodged in the brain of sheep, the first signs will be shown in about eight to twelve days. Bladder worms produce a congestion of the brain which causes dullness, dizziness, indicating an affection of the brain, walking or turning in circles. If the left side of the brain is affected they will turn to the left; if the right side is affected, they will turn to the right. The head eventually droops, the eyes become red and the vision is impaired, the head very hot over the affected region, the affected sheep become separated from the flock. Sometimes the sheep are partially or completely paralyzed.

PREVENTION: Prevention is the only method by which this disease can be eradicated. Prevent the sheep from becoming infected with these parasites. Stray dogs, wolves or coyotes should be killed whenever found, and dogs too valuable to kill should be kept free from tapeworm. Meat should not be fed to dogs unless cooked or known to be free from tapeworm cysts.

GRUBS IN THE HEAD

(Head Maggot)

CAUSE: Grubs in the head of sheep are produced by the Sheep Gadfly which is yellowish-gray in color with five well divided rings around its body, covered over with fine hair and the lower portion of the head white. This fly is somewhat larger than the ordinary house fly. It attacks sheep and goats during the Summer and Fall and deposits its larva about the sheep's and goat's nostrils. This larva attaches itself to the mucous membrane of the nostrils with two hooklets by which it gradually works into the air cavities of the head, remaining there for about ten months. Then it again passes from the nostrils, burrows into the ground and becomes a fully matured Gadfly in six or eight weeks, which completes its life cycle, the head of the sheep or goat being its intermediate host where the newly born Gadfly again attaches its larva.

SYMPTOMS: When sheep or goats are attacked by this Gadfly, they run, strike at the nose with their front feet, rub the nose on the ground or against other sheep. In case only three or four larvae gain entrance to the sinuses of the head, they produce very little, if any, ill effects, but where they become numerous, they cause the animal to cough and sneeze continually, discharge from the nose, which is occasionally tinged with blood. The appetite becomes impaired, the animal shows signs of emaciation, becomes very weak, raises the nose in the air, but eventually becomes so weak it reels when walking and finally lies down. It becomes so weak it cannot toss the head or rise, and dies.

PREVENTION TREATMENT: Very successful. Paint the sheep's or goat's nose with Pine Tar, or better still, place salt in a trough, covering it with boards, with holes bored in them just large enough for the animal to insert its nose. Smear Pine Tar about the holes once or twice a week. This treatment has proven very efficient in localities where sheep Gadflies are numerous.

MEDICAL TREATMENT: After the animal once becomes infected with these grubs, bore holes (trephine) through the skull with a sharp instrument made for this purpose and remove the grubs. This requires considerable amount of skill and should be attempted only by a competent Veterinarian.

HOVEN

(Bloating--Acute Tynpanitis--Acute Indigestion)

CAUSE: Hoven is caused by various kinds of food which produce indigestion or fermentation and resultant gases in the rumen or paunch. When sheep are first turned into young clover, they eat so greedily of it that bloating frequently results. Turnips, potatoes and cabbage may also produce it. Middlings and corn meal also frequently give rise to it. In this connection it may be stated that an excessive quantity of any food, before mentioned, may bring on this disorder, or it may not be due to excessive eating but to eating too fast. Sometimes the quality of food is at fault. Grass, clover or alfalfa, when wet with dew or rain soaked, frequently produce digestive disorders and bloating follows. Frozen roots or potatoes covered with white frost should be regarded as dangerous. When food has been eaten too hastily or when it is cold and wet, the digestive process is imperfectly performed and the food contained in the paunch ferments, during which process large quantities of gas are formed. This same result may follow when a sheep is choking, as the obstruction in the gullet prevents the eructation or passing of gas from the stomach so that the gas continues to accumulate until severe bloating results.

SYMPTOMS: The swelling of the left flank is very characteristic, as in well marked cases the flank at its upper part rises above the level of the backbone and when struck with the tips of the fingers emits a drum-like sound. The animal has an anxious expression, moves uneasily and is evidently distressed. If relief is not obtained in time the sheep breathes with difficulty, reels in walking or standing and in a short time falls down and dies from suffocation. The distention of the stomach or rumen may become so great that it pushes the diaphragm (the membrane separating the lung and intestinal cavity) forward against the lungs, so as to squeeze and stop their movements, thus preventing the animal from breathing and in some instances the case may be complicated by a rupture of the stomach.

TREATMENT: Do not waste any time. Puncture about three inches downward and forward from the point of the hip bone with a clean sharp knife, or any instrument that is clean and sharp. A special instrument made for this purpose, the trocar, is a very useful instrument on the farm.

Sometimes bloating becomes chronic, and if such is the case dissolve two teaspoonfuls of Turpentine in one-half pint of milk and drench the animal very carefully, as some of this drench may escape into the lungs and produce fatal pneumonia. Set a sheep upon its haunches to give the medicine; if it coughs let it down quickly to prevent strangulation.

INDIGESTION

(Dyspepsia)

CAUSE: Irritant food, damaged food, overloaded paunch or sudden change of diet may produce this disease. Want of exercise predisposes an animal to it and it is caused by woody or indigestible food. Food which possesses astringent (drying) properties tends to check the digestive secretions and may also act as an exciting cause. Food in excessive quantity may lead to disorders of the digestion and to this disease. It is very likely to appear towards the end of the protracted season of draught, therefore a deficiency of water must be regarded as one of the conditions which favors its development.

SYMPTOMS: Appetite diminished; rumination, or chewing the cud, irregular; tongue coated, mouth slimy, feces passed apparently not well digested and offensive in odor, dullness and fullness of the flanks. This disease may, in some cases, assume a chronic character, for in addition to the above mentioned symptoms, slight bloating of the left flank may be observed. The animal breathes with great difficulty and grunts with each respiration. The ears and legs alternately become hot and cold. The rumination, or cud chewing, at this stage ceases and the usual rumbling sound in the stomach is not audible. The passage of feces is entirely suspended and the animal passes only a little mucus occasionally. Sometimes constipation and diarrhoea alternate; there is a rise in temperature in many cases. The disease continues for a few days or a week in this mild form, while the severe form of the disease may last for several weeks. In the severe form the emaciation and loss of strength may be very great. There is no appetite, no rumination or rumbling sound in the stomach or intestines. The mouth is hot and sticky, the eyes have retracted in their sockets and the milk secretion has ceased. In such cases the outlook for recovery is unfavorable. The affected animals fall away in flesh and become very weak, which is shown by the fact that one finds the animal lying down.

On examination of sheep or goats which have died of this disease, it is found that the lining membranes of the fourth stomach and intestines, particularly the small intestines, are red, swollen, streaked with deep red or blushed lines or spotted. The lining of the third stomach is more or less softened and may be easily pealed off. The third stomach contains dry, hard food masses, closely adhering to its walls. In some cases the brain appears to become affected, probably from the pain endured and weakness and absorption of poisons generated in the digestive canal. In such cases there is weakness and a staggering gait; the sheep or goats do not appear to see, and will consequently run against obstacles. After a time it falls down and gives up to a violent disordered struggle. This delirious condition is succeeded by stupor and death.

TREATMENT: Successful; if fed in its first stages on small quantities of roots, sweet silage or select grasses or hay. This should be offered several times daily. Very little food should be allowed if the animal is constipated, in which case give two to four ounces of Glauber Salts dissolved in a pint of hot water. When it cools, set the animal on its haunches and pour slowly and carefully. If they strangle or cough let them down, as some of the drench may escape into the lungs and produce lung complications. After the Glauber Salts have acted and if there is a lack of appetite and the animal does not chew the cud regularly, the following tonic will be found beneficial: Pulv. Gentian Root, one ounce; Pulv. Nux Vomica, one ounce; Pulv. Anise Seed, two ounces. Mix thoroughly and make into thirty-two powders. Give one powder two or three times a day well back on the tongue. The food must be rather laxative and of a digestible character. After an attack of this form of indigestion, ice cold water should be avoided. Food should be given in moderate quantities, as any excess by overtaxing the digestive functions may bring on a relapse.

JAUNDICE

(Liver Congestion--Inflammation of the Liver)

CAUSE: Jaundice or Liver Congestion is due to constipation where there is an inactive or torpid condition of the bowels and the bile which passes into the intestines is absorbed and produces a yellow staining of Jaundice. Jaundice is merely a symptom of a disease and ought to direct attention to ascertain if possible the cause or causes which give rise to it. Inflammation of the liver usually occurs as a complication of infectious diseases. It may also occur as a complication of intestinal catarrh, or in hot weather from overheating, eating decomposed or irritating food or from drinking stagnant water.

SYMPTOMS: The signs are sometimes obscure and their real significance is frequently overlooked. The most prominent symptoms are the yellowness of the white of the eyes and of the mucous membranes lining the mouth, appetite poor, body presents an emaciated appearance, the feces is light in color, while the urine is likely to be unusually dark and there is great thirst present. The gait is weak and the animal lies down more than usual and while doing so frequently has its head around resting on the side of its chest. Temperature is slightly elevated above normal and breathing is somewhat hurried.

TREATMENT: Remove the cause if possible. Give Glauber Salts in three to four ounce doses, diluted in a pint of hot water permitted to cool and give at one dose. When drenching be very careful, as some of the liquid may escape into the lungs and produce severe complications. Feed green food or hot bran mashes and supply them with a liberal quantity of pure water to drink.

LIVER FLUKE

CAUSE: The parasite that produces Liver Fluke in sheep has an oblong, flat, leaf-like body, brownish in color, measuring from one-fourth to one-half inch in length. Sheep become infected with this Liver Fluke from grazing on low marshy pastures infected by the larvae of Liver Fluke.

SYMPTOMS: A sheep, when first infected with Liver Fluke, generally thrives as the parasites tend to stimulate the process of digestion, being located as they are in the liver, but eventually rumination becomes irregular, the sheep becomes anemic, weak and the visible mucous membranes of the mouth, nose and eyes become pale, bloodless, taking on a yellowish color as the disease progresses. Swellings will also appear under the jaw along the neck and under the lung cavity. The process of breathing becomes feeble and temperature irregular. Pregnant ewes will generally abort and nursing ewes' milk will become so deprived of its nourishing properties that the lambs become emaciated, although not necessarily affected with the Liver Fluke.

PREVENTION: Move to non-infected pastures, supply the animals grazing on low marshy pastures with a liberal amount of salt, also introduce frogs, toads, carp, etc., into the marshy ponds, as they destroy the parasite in its first stages of development, feeding on their intermediate host, the snail.

MEDICAL TREATMENT: This is of little value. After an animal once becomes infected with the parasite, it never makes a complete recovery, although Calomel administered in ten grain doses every two or three weeks appears to have a very good effect in some cases, if fed freely on nitrogenous food and permitted to drink well of pure running water.

LUNG FEVER

(Pneumonia--Congestion of the Lungs--Pulmonary Apoplexy)

Acute congestion and inflammation of the spongy tissues of the lungs is frequently seen in sheep, the same as in other animals.

CAUSE: Sheep that are over driven are subject to Lung Congestion in acute or chronic form and sometimes Pulmonary Apoplexy, and especially when in a plethoric condition are predisposed to inflammation of the lungs. The exciting cause is very much the same as in different diseases of the air passage and it is not uncommon for the inflammation to extend from these parts of the lungs. However, there are a number of causes in addition to those already mentioned. It frequently results when sheep are accustomed to warm, comfortable quarters and are changed to cold, drafty pens, or shipping some distance in open stock cars during cold weather. In fact, any sudden chilling of the body is a common cause of lung disorders. Giving fat sheep too much exercise when they are not accustomed to it is a very frequent cause of Congestion and Inflammation of the Lungs. This may occur when they are chased by dogs, etc., or when driven to a distant market at too rapid a gait. Exercise during the hot summer months is apt to cause congestion of the lung substance, as well as heat stroke. Dipping sheep during cold weather may chill the body and result in this disease.

SYMPTOMS: If due to severe exercise, the animal appears greatly exhausted and the Congestion of the Lungs is marked. Death may occur in this stage of the disease. Inflammation of the Lungs usually begins with a chill and is followed by a high fever. The sheep stand most of the time and may eat nothing, or very little. The breathing is hurried at first, but when the lungs become badly involved, it is also labored. The character of the pulse beats varies, depending on the extent of the inflammation and the stage of the disease. In most cases the pulse is full and quick during the early stages of the disease. A very weak pulse is present in severe and fatal cases of Pneumonia. The visible mucous membranes have a red colored appearance and there may be a slight discharge from the nostrils. The expression of the face is anxious and distressed in severe cases and rigors and chilling of the body occur. The respiratory sounds are more or less normal. The cough at first is deep and dry; later it becomes loose and moist. It may be accompanied by a hemorrhage during this stage of the disease. Other respiratory sounds are revealed by placing the ear to the side of the chest walls and listening to the sound of the lungs. This cannot be practiced in long wooled sheep with satisfaction, as the chest walls are so thick that the lung sounds are deadened, or the noise made by the animal hides the respiratory murmurs in the very early stages of Inflammation of the Lungs. A crepitating or crackling sound can be heard in the diseased parts and louder sounds than normal in the healthy areas. Later when the engorgement of the lung substance occurs and the air cells become filled with an inflammatory serum, the respiratory sounds are deadened, but on returning to the normal, a rattling sound occurs. These symptoms help greatly in determining the animal's condition and in watching the progress of the disease. The chances for the recovery depend on the extent and the acuteness of the inflammation. Careless handling, exercising, etc., lessen the chances for a favorable termination in the disease, but good care helps more to bring about recovery than the medical treatment. The recovery is more unfavorable in fat than in lean sheep, as the inflammation is usually more severe in the former. The course is from seven to twenty-one days and it may become chronic if the irritation is kept up. In such cases, unthriftiness is a prominent sign.

TREATMENT: The preventive treatment in Pneumonia must not be overlooked. Briefly, it consists in avoiding such conditions as may predispose the animal to the disease or act in any way as an exciting cause. Careful nursing is a very important part of the treatment. The sheep should be given a comfortable, well ventilated shed and kept as quiet as possible. If the bowels become constipated, give two or three ounces of Castor Oil and feed sloppy food. As one attack predisposes the sheep to a second, it should be protected from severe cold, or the other extreme, heat, for a month after making a complete recovery.

The following prescription will be found very beneficial: Iodide of Ammonia, one-half ounce; Chlorate of Potassi, one ounce; Pulv. Nux Vomica, one ounce. Make into twenty-four powders and give one powder every four hours well back on the tongue. Continue this treatment until the animal has recovered.

LUNG WORMS, LAMB DISEASE

(Verminous Bronchitis)

CAUSE: Due to a white thread-like worm (Strongylus Filaria) varying in length from one to three inches. These worms affect and live in the trachea (windpipe) and bronchial tubes. Infected animals, in coughing, expel fertilized eggs which develop on the grass and stagnant water. The larvae are again taken up either in the drinking water or in eating grass or hay gathered on low marshy soil. Warm wet weather favors their development.

SYMPTOMS: This worm is liable to attack a number of animals at the same time. The weakest sheep and young lambs are the first to show signs by coughing forcibly, distressing, hacking and convulsive in character. A stringy mucus is sometimes expelled during the spasm of coughing. This mucus contains worms which can be detected, or their ova observed under a magnifying glass. In the latter stages of the disease, they cough severely at night. These attacks have a sub-acute character and prove very exhausting. The parasite by becoming entwined in balls severely affects the animal's breathing which is always remarkably labored in the latter stages of the disease. The animal refuses to eat, becomes emaciated, anemic, mucous membranes of the eyes, mouth and nose become very pale and the sheep die in convulsions from suffocation.

PREVENTIVE TREATMENT: Avoid grazing your sheep on low marshy soil, especially during warm wet weather. Young lambs and weak ewes are especially susceptible to this disease.

MEDICAL TREATMENT: The writer has tried various treatments as fumigation with different substances and injection of remedies into the windpipe by the use of a hypodermic syringe, etc., but none have proven very successful, from a practical standpoint. I would recommend placing the affected animals in a tightly closed barn or shed, in the center of which place a pan of red hot coals and cover with Sulphur.

A person should remain in the barn or shed as long as he possibly can and after the fumes become so irritating that he cannot endure them any longer, he should immediately make his exit. The sheep should be compelled to stay a minute or two longer and then quickly open the doors and windows. Repeat this treatment once or twice a week. Feed affected animals well. Give them fresh water to drink and protect them from exposure. This treatment, as above described, has given very good results, providing the parasites were not too numerous.

SCAB

(Mange)

CAUSE: The mange mite (Psoroptes Communis). This parasite is equipped with stylets which pierce the skin at the seat where the mange mite penetrates the skin, and produces small red spots followed by a blister filled with serum, which ruptures, the serum drying and forming a small scab. It is in this way that innumerable mange mites cause the piling up of scabs thus producing a very scaly condition. As Mange advances, the scaly patches eventually pile up until they attain the thickness of one-half inch, unless these scabs have been severely rubbed.

SYMPTOMS: Very easily detected, as a bunch of sheep that have been recently infected will be uneasy or restless, rubbing, against fences, posts, brush, etc., causing bunches of wool to loosen. The itching seems to be more intense at night and during warm weather. The affected animals will even make attempts to bite themselves, due to the agony produced by the mange mite. If the skin is examined by the aid of a magnifying glass, the mange mite can be easily noticed, or by scraping the skin with a knife and placing the scabs on a dark paper and exposed to the warmth of the sun, the mange mite moving about can readily be seen with the naked eye. Mangy sheep become very poor and eventually die.

PREVENTION: This is important, for although the disease is treated with very good results, the mange mite annoy the sheep until they become very weak and emaciated and the loss of wool is enormous due to the affected animal continually rubbing against fences, brush, etc.

TREATMENT: Consists of using various dips, as Lime and Sulphur, which is recommended by the United States Bureau of Animal Industry. This is very effective and inexpensive. Scabby sheep should be dipped a week or ten days after shearing; two dippings are necessary at the interval of ten days. After dipping, move to non-infected range or pastures.

TICK

(Louse Fly)

CAUSE: The tick that infects sheep has a very small head sunken into its round body. The head possesses a flexible trunk or snout that penetrates the skin. Through this trunk, the ticks derive their nourishment by sucking the blood from the body of the sheep. The tick is also provided with three pairs of legs. The female lays her young in the form of a spun egg (cocoon) which is oblong in shape and brown in color. This egg is cemented to the wool of sheep where young ticks are hatched in about four to six weeks.

SYMPTOMS: Long wooled sheep are more susceptible to this tick as their wool provides shelter for both the tick and its eggs. After shearing the sheep the ticks have a tendency to leave the body and to migrate to the legs or to unshorn lambs where their snouts or trunks pierce the skin which appears to become infected, producing a swelling and inflammation. The infected sheep run, scratch and bite themselves. When these ticks become developed in large quantities, they produce a paleness of the mucous membranes of the eyes, mouth and nose, as the ticks suck large quantities of blood, which produces an anemic condition. The sheep become poor, weak and unthrifty.

TREATMENT: Satisfactorily treated by dipping infected sheep in Coal Tar dips or Emulsions of Crude Petroleum. Shearing the sheep has a good effect, but care must be exercised as the ticks then rapidly migrate to the lambs.

DISEASES OF POULTRY

Causes, Symptoms and Treatments

CHAPTER V

AIR SAC MITE

CAUSE: Produced by a parasite called Cylodites Nudus, which bears a close resemblance to the parasite causing mange or scabies in the domesticated animal. Owing to the peculiar construction of their breathing organs fowls are more susceptible to parasites than animals. In addition to affecting the lungs, the Air Sac Mite may extend its operations to the intestines, kidneys, liver and bones.

SYMPTOMS: Unthriftiness is first noticed, but after the parasites become numerous, the fowl shows signs of difficult breathing, perhaps terminating in bronchial pneumonia. In some cases death occurs without apparent cause. The bird will be inactive, becomes separated from the rest of the flock, comb pale, head drawn close to the body, wings hang pendulous, lose flesh, breathing becomes hard, coughing, sneezing and a rattling from the mucus in the windpipe is heard. Death is produced from suffocation.

TREATMENT: Separate the sick from the healthy fowls. Disinfect coops and runways of both sick and healthy birds with Crude Carbolic Acid, undiluted. Also fumigate the fowls in their coops with steam from hot water and Pine Tar. This may be done by placing the water and Tar in a pan and then inserting a hot stone or brick in the solution. This perhaps is the simplest method of fumigation. Also mix Sulphur in their feed regularly.

APOPLEXY

(Hemorrhage of the Brain)

Due to the rupture of a blood vessel of the brain and pressure from the escaping blood.

CAUSE: Mechanical injuries, straining when laying eggs (hens are frequently found dead on the nest from this cause), overfeeding, stimulating food, etc., all tend to produce apoplexy.

SYMPTOMS: Appear very suddenly, bird is seen to walk unsteadily, falls, or perhaps is found dead.

TREATMENT: In mild attacks, apply cold water or ice to fowl's head until thoroughly cooled. Give one-half grain of Calomel, feed soft food, compel the bird to exercise. Owing to the loss of blood a tonic will be necessary. Pulv. Gentian Root, Pulv. Saltpeter, Capsicum and Ferri Sulphate (Pulv.) equal parts one ounce. Mix and place one teaspoonful in feed for every twenty-five fowls. This tonic purifies and builds up the blood, just what is needed in this particular condition.

BALDNESS

(Favus)

CAUSE: Due to fungi.

SYMPTOMS: The first noticeable sign is the whitish appearance of the comb due to gray spots about the size of a pin head. As the disease progresses, this condition spreads to other parts of the body; the feathers look rough and dry and break easily. The fowl grows weaker, refuses to eat and if not properly treated, dies.

TREATMENT: Remove the scabs by separating the feathers and using a brush. Apply Sulphur Ointment. Repeat this treatment after two or three days. Great care must be taken to prevent the fowl from chilling or taking cold.

BEAK AND THROAT OBSTRUCTION

CAUSE: Lodgment in the beak or food canal of a foreign substance, such as a kernel of corn, sunflower seed, bone, etc.

SYMPTOMS: Fowl jerks its head suddenly and frequently attempts to swallow. If a close examination is made the foreign body can be felt from the outside.

TREATMENT: For the removal of such obstructions, no special treatment is needed further than to use care and avoid any injury to the beak or throat. Feed nutritious food, as wheat bran mashes and vegetables and see that they have a liberal quantity of good pure water at all times.

BLACKHEAD

(Infectious Entero Hepatitis of Turkeys)

CAUSE: Due to a protozoa taken into the system with the food or drinking water. This parasite enters the caeca which becomes inflamed and discolored and the liver is enlarged and studded with yellowish spots about the size of a pea.

SYMPTOMS: Although this disease is termed Blackhead, the discoloration of the head is not necessarily present in all cases; neither is this condition confined to this particular disease. One of the first symptoms is loss of appetite, followed in most cases by diarrhoea. The fowl becomes weak and loses weight rapidly. Examination of the liver after death will determine whether or not death has been caused by Infectious Entero Hepatitis. The dead birds should be burned to prevent the spread of the disease.

TREATMENT: Prevention is one of the most important factors as this disease is very contagious and the protozoa once implanted in the turkey runs is almost impossible to eradicate. Provide clean, well ventilated coops and feed clean, wholesome food and good fresh water to drink.

MEDICAL TREATMENT: Give Bismuth Salicylate and Quinine Sulphate each one grain two to three times a day. Also mix Hyposulphite of Soda in the proportion of two to four grains to every fowl in their drinking water twice daily. Disinfect coops and runs with Crude Carbolic Acid, undiluted.

BODY LICE

CAUSE: Insanitary conditions. Communicated by direct contact.

SYMPTOMS: Young chicks become emaciated and die quickly. Older birds withstand the parasite much longer, but in time show signs of uneasiness by dusting themselves frequently. The comb and wattles become pale and bloodless, the feathers rough, dry and brittle. The birds grow weak, poor, and eventually die.

TREATMENT: Dust the birds with the following: Sulphur, one part; Napthaline, one part; Tobacco Dust, twenty-eight parts and seventy parts of middlings. Powder finely and mix well together and dust the birds once daily. Also sprinkle freely in the dust baths.

BRONCHITIS

CAUSE: Exposure to dampness, cold drafts of air, inhaling irritating gases, vapors or dust. The fowls should be carefully examined, as bronchitis is occasionally caused by the presence of gapeworms.

SYMPTOMS: Loss of appetite, the bird moves about slowly, breathing with difficulty and making a sort of whistling sound accompanied by a cough. As the disease progresses, there will be a peculiar bubbling sound from breathing due to an excessive accumulation of mucus in the windpipe. At this stage of the disease the bird becomes very weak and if not properly treated and cared for will rapidly lose strength, the feathers will become rough, head and wings droop, and the bird dies.

TREATMENT: This disease is most satisfactorily treated by placing the affected birds in warm, dry, well ventilated quarters, admitting sunlight if possible, but excluding all drafts of air. Feed stale bread, middlings, etc. Also place the fowls in a moderately air tight coop and compel them to inhale steam from hot water and Turpentine. This is readily done by placing the water and Turpentine in a pan and then insert a hot stone or brick in the solution. Force them to inhale this steam from twenty to thirty minutes twice a day. Also add Chlorate of Potash to their drinking water, one teaspoonful to every twenty-five aged fowls. To chicks add one-fourth teaspoonful to every twenty-five. If the weather is favorable and the above treatment is followed, bronchitis yields very favorably.

BUMBLE FOOT

(Corns-Deep Bruises-Abscesses)

CAUSE: Sharp-edged or narrow perches which bruise the feet or where the perches are high, heavy fowls often injure their feet by alighting on stones or other hard objects.

SYMPTOMS: The bird limps or hobbles about, moving with great difficulty. Examination will show the foot to be hot and tender to the touch.

TREATMENT: Wash with clean, warm water and in some cases it is advisable to apply Hot Flaxseed poultices. When soft spots or abscesses develop, lance them with a clean, sharp knife. After abscesses and bruises are opened, treat them antiseptically by washing with a solution of Carbolic Acid, one teaspoonful to a pint of water. The foot should be bandaged to keep out dust and dirt.

CATARRH

CAUSE: Exposure; poorly constructed coops which admit rain or drafts. Weak birds are very susceptible to Catarrh.

SYMPTOMS: The bird is dull, moves about slowly, coughing or sneezing; appetite is poor, the mucous membrane of the air passage becomes inflamed and the breathing difficult, especially through the nose. The discharge from the nostrils at first watery, becomes mucus-like and thick and sticky, closing the nose, causing the bird to breathe wholly through the mouth with a wheezing sound.

TREATMENT: The cause of Catarrh shows the necessity of clean and comfortable quarters for the fowls. Keep the birds strong and vigorous by feeding clean, nourishing food.

MEDICAL TREATMENT: To each fowl administer in their drinking water or feed: Chlorate of Potash, one grain, twice daily.

CHICKEN POX

(Sore Head--Warts)

CAUSE: These diseases are due to low forms of parasites or fungi and occur most frequently in wet weather especially if the coops are leaky and allow the rain to fall on the droppings, causing mold or fungi. Poor ventilation and lack of light also promotes the growth of fungi.

SYMPTOMS: The disease is usually confined to the head and affects principally young chickens, pigeons and turkeys, but rarely ducks and geese. The infection appears in the form of yellowish warts or nodules about the nose, eyelids, comb, wattles, under the wings, or any unfeathered place. The warts vary in size from that of a pin head to the size of a pea and they discharge a fluid which at first is thin and watery but as the disease progresses, it becomes thick and sticky, yellow in color and fetid in smell. At this stage the appetite is poor, the feathers appear rough, and where the eyelids are affected, as in most cases, the bird cannot see, fails to eat, becomes emaciated, loses weight and strength rapidly and if not properly treated, dies.

TREATMENT: This disease is very contagious, therefore the coops and runs should be disinfected with Crude Carbolic Acid, undiluted. In the drinking water add Hyposulphite of Soda in the proportion of one to two grains to each fowl (one-half grain to chicks). Wash the nodules or warts about the head with Carbolic Acid solution, one teaspoonful to a quart of water. Feed easily digested food, such as vegetables or warm bran mashes.

CONGESTION OF THE LIVER

CAUSE: Lack of exercise, overfeeding, tainted or moldy food, infection, or impure blood.

SYMPTOMS: Birds suffering from this disease seldom show signs of sickness and it is well to dissect the fowl after death to ascertain the exact cause. If death is caused by Congestion of the Liver, the organ will be greatly enlarged and easily torn.

TREATMENT: If the fowls are fat and sluggish, compel them to exercise by driving them about. Also give fifteen to twenty grains of Epsom Salts to each affected fowl. Feed laxative foods that are easily digested, as vegetables and wheat bran mashes. They are cooling and relieve congestion.

CONGESTION OF THE LUNGS

(Pulmonary Congestion)

CAUSE: Exposure; the bird chills, causing contraction of the blood vessels near the surface of the body, thereby forcing a large quantity of blood to the internal organs; the small blood vessels in the lungs become distended with blood and rupture.

SYMPTOMS: Rapid and difficult breathing; the bird appears stupid and sleepy and docs not care to move about; appetite poor, wings drooping, plumage ruffled, a thick mucus, colored with blood, escapes from the mouth, comb and wattles show a dark-red color from lack of oxygen in the blood. This disease is of very short duration, the bird dying within a few hours. It is very common among young chicks and turkeys that are permitted to run out in the early spring rains.

TREATMENT: Medical treatment is of no value, as the disease progresses so rapidly that the bird dies shortly after the first symptoms appear. Sanitary surroundings, good light, pure air and exercise are essential. Do not allow the birds to stand out in the cold or rains, especially during the molting season. Keep your poultry strong and vigorous by feeding clean, nourishing food and give them pure water to drink.

CONSTIPATION

(Intestinal Obstruction)

CAUSE: Irritation of the membranes lining the intestines, caused by dry feed, glass or gravel; may also be due to parasitic worms. Obstruction may occur in any part of the intestines although the external opening is the part most frequently affected.

SYMPTOMS: Bird appears dull and stupid, walks with difficulty and attempts frequently to expel the obstructing material. The appetite is poor and the feathers rough. By examination and manipulation the obstruction may be located. Dried masses of excrement by adhering to the feathers sometimes block the outer opening of the intestines.

TREATMENT: Remove the waste matter clinging to the feathers with warm water or by clipping the feathers off. If the Cloaca is obstructed, give injections of Sweet Oil or Olive Oil with a small bulb syringe. Also give one to two grains of Calomel and feed clean food and soft mashes containing Pulv. Gentian Root, one grain to each fowl twice daily. This stimulates the worm-like movement of the bowels and assists in expelling their contents.

CROP IMPACTION

(Obstruction, Paralysis, Inflammation, Catarrh)

CAUSE: Errors in feeding; birds that are not fed regularly are predisposed to any of the above conditions; may also be due to swallowing large pieces of bone, thread, nails, pins, glass, gravel, etc.

SYMPTOMS: Loss of appetite, frequent attempts to swallow, crop greatly distended and hard on pressure; eventually the food decomposes and a liquid may escape from the mouth and nose. The bird appears dull, stupid and sleepy, comb pale, feathers rough, beak open, owing to pressure on the windpipe. If caused by swallowing sharp objects, they may penetrate the crop and skin, causing a gangrenous condition. Grain in the crop will sometimes send out sprouts of considerable lengths.

TREATMENT: If no sharp objects are present, give two teaspoonfuls of Sweet or Olive Oil. This will lubricate the esophagus and crop. Manipulate the crop upward, forcing the food gently through the mouth, adding oil occasionally. If, however, sharp objects penetrate the crop it is best to remove them through an artificial opening. Clip the feathers from around the intended seat of operation and wash the clipped surface with a Carbolic Solution, one teaspoonful to a pint of water. The incision should not be over one-half inch long and should be made as high as possible and in the center of the crop. After removing the contents, sew up with ordinary thread and needle and wash occasionally with the above antiseptic solution. The operation is not difficult and will be successful if the parts are not too badly inflamed.

After-treatment consists of feeding very little food until the crop is fairly well healed. Feed soft bran mashes and vegetables. To the drinking water add Boracic Acid, one grain, twice daily. It relieves the catarrhal condition that is present, such as irritations of the crop and intestines.

DIARRHOEA

(Gastro-Intestinal Catarrh--Enteritis)

CAUSE: Inflammation of the digestive organs can be traced in every instance to the quality or quantity of food and water consumed. The food or water may contain parasites, or large quantities of mustard, pepper, or may be moldy or tainted.

SYMPTOMS: Loss of appetite, the feathers appear rough, the crop is sometimes paralyzed and distended with gas, the bird moves slowly, the droppings vary in color from a white to a yellow or a green and finally becomes tinged with blood; at this stage there is a rise in temperature accompanied by great thirst and signs of pain. Mild cases of simple diarrhoea if not properly treated when first symptoms appear, will develop the same severe conditions described above.

TREATMENT: Determine the cause and remove it if possible. See that the food is clean and nutritious, the coops well ventilated, the runs well lighted. Sunlight is very beneficial. Avoid exposure, drafts and dampness. Place oatmeal in their drinking water, also give two grains of Bismuth mixed with dough and make into a small pill. Give one every six hours.

When in addition to the above symptoms a bloody discharge is present, give six drops of Tincture of Catechu every four hours. Warm mashes made of bran or oatmeal are very nourishing and soothing to the intestinal canal.

DIPHTHERITIC ROUP

(Diphtheria)

CAUSE: Due to a specific germ. The disease is very contagious and is communicated by direct contact. Great care should be exercised, therefore, when showing or buying birds. Any new birds to be added to the flock should be kept in separate pens for a week or two to make sure they are in good condition.

SYMPTOMS: The first symptoms are similar to those of catarrh or cold. A clear, watery liquid escapes from the eyes and nostrils, the head is drawn in toward the body, the feathers appear rough, the breathing fast, the temperature rises from three to five degrees above normal. The bird walks about as if blind, sneezing, swallowing with difficulty, and showing signs of great weakness. If the mouth is opened small white spots or elevations will be seen on the back of the tongue. There may be diarrhoea of a green or yellow color. As the disease progresses the discharge from the nose and eyes becomes thick and stringy, obstructing the air passages and gathering in large quantities between the eyelids. The mouth, throat and tongue are very much inflamed and swollen and in most cases it is impossible for the bird to make a sound. Recovery is doubtful after the disease has reached this stage.

TREATMENT: Isolate the affected birds in some clean, warm, light, well ventilated quarters, excluding drafts. Dissolve thirty grains of Chlorate of Potash in one ounce of water and one ounce of Glycerine, and to the average sized fowl give one teaspoonful three or four times a day. To chicks give one-fourth the dose. When the scum loosens in the back part of the tongue, remove the scum gently, Care should be taken so as to prevent bleeding. Feed soft, nourishing food.

DOUBLE-YOLK EGGS

Eggs are frequently found with two yolks. This condition is produced by two ovary capsules bursting at about the same time and gaining entrance together into the oviduct where they are concealed in the same shell. Double-yolked eggs are larger than normal and may injure the oviduct when expelled. When hatched, they produce twins or abnormal chicks.

DROPSY

(Ascites)

CAUSE: Generally due to irritating, indigestible food, causing inflammation of the membranous lining of the intestinal cavity.

SYMPTOMS: The abdomen becomes enlarged, is tender to the touch and contains a watery fluid, the movement of which can be heard in most cases by pressure on the swollen parts. The bird appears stupid, the comb pale and the appetite poor.

TREATMENT: Unless the bird is very valuable, treatment is not advisable. In case the bird is valuable, give one grain of Potassium Iodide twice daily in the feed or drinking water. Also feed nourishing food as beef-scraps, vegetables, wheat bran mashes, etc.

EGG BOUND

(Difficult Laying; Obstruction of the Oviduct)

CAUSE: Due to the eggs being too large, the bird too fat, or to the absence of the secretions lubricating the oviduct.

SYMPTOMS: The first signs are scarcely noticeable but soon the feathers appear rough, the bird becomes dull and moves slowly, making frequent efforts to expel the egg.

TREATMENT: Remove the egg by injecting Sweet Oil, assisting the bird with gentle pressure. In some cases it is well to puncture the egg and collapse the shell. If the bird is very fat, reduce by careful feeding. If the bird is of normal size, the trouble is probably due to the absence of lubricating secretions of the oviduct, in which case the following tonic should be given: Pulv. Ferri Sulphate, Pulv. Gentian Root, each one dram. Mix and make into thirty powders. Give one powder two or three times a day in their feed for a week or ten days.

EGG EATING

CAUSE: Is usually due to lack of shell-building material in the food; in such case the shell of the egg is thin and easily broken and the fowl craving the lime contained in the egg shell, naturally contracts the habit.

TREATMENT: Supply ground bone and oyster shells. Feed green food such as cabbage, kale, potatoes, carrots, etc.

EGGS WITHOUT SHELLS

(Soft-Shelled Eggs)

CAUSE: Deficiency of shell material; or it is possible that fright sometimes causes premature expulsion of the eggs before the shell is formed.

TREATMENT: Feed ground bone, oyster shells. They contain egg shell producing material. Perhaps the best results are obtained when mixed with wheat bran. Also feed vegetables such as cabbage, potatoes and carrots.

FEATHER PULLING

(Feather Eating)

CAUSE: Irritation of the skin due to lice, mites or to lack of exercise and improper food.

TREATMENT: Feed meat, ground bones and vegetables. Place the food where the fowls are compelled to scratch and work to obtain it. Dust the fowls with Powdered Aloes.

If due to lice, treat the same as recommended under the heading of Lice.

GAPES

(Verminous Tracheo Bronchitis)

CAUSE: A red, parasitic worm, the male measuring about one-fifth of an inch and the female one-half an inch in length. Fowls become infected by eating worms containing this parasite or its eggs, and by coming in contact with other birds suffering from the disease.

SYMPTOMS: The most noticeable symptom is frequent gaping; the Gapeworms attach themselves by their months to the walls of the windpipe where they suck the blood which nourishes them; they cause irritation and inflammation of the windpipe, bronchial tubes and lungs; breathing is difficult and the bird loses strength rapidly; windpipe eventually becomes totally obstructed and the bird dies from suffocation and exhaustion. Young, weak chickens are more susceptible to this disease than strong ones.

TREATMENT: Separate the sick birds from the healthy ones. Clean and disinfect the coops and runs. Burn all manure. Remove the worms from the windpipe by the use of a feather, from which the fan has been stripped, leaving only a small brush at the end. Dip the feather into Oil of Turpentine or Coal Oil, removing the surplus liquid by drawing the feather between the fingers. Now insert the feather into the windpipe of the bird and by turning gently you will dislodge the worms from their attachments. Repeat this treatment once a day for two or three days. Disinfect coops and runs with undiluted Crude Carbolic Acid. Feed good nutritious food as wheat bran mashes, etc.

HEAD LICE

CAUSE: Result of insanitary conditions and lack of care. Communicated by direct contact with infected birds, or by infected coops or brooders.

SYMPTOMS: The head soon becomes denuded of feathers, and also sore by being constantly scratched with the feet. If not properly treated the chicks weaken and die.

TREATMENT: An ointment made of one part Sulphur and four parts Lard well mixed and applied two to three times will exterminate the lice. If the fowl is run down in condition, feed good nutritious food as wheat bran mashes.

HOW TO FEED YOUNG POULTRY

Withhold all food for at least eighteen hours; then feed stale bread moistened with boiled milk every three hours. When they are three or four days old, feed rolled oats, ground corn moistened with pure water, finely chopped meat and boiled vegetables. Feed them often and you will be well repaid by their rapid growth, strength, and the low death rate. After they reach the age of one week or ten days, watch them closely and regulate their feed to their apparent needs.

INCOMPLETE EGG

(Abortion)

CAUSE: Irritation of the oviduct; improper secretion of albumen or internal egg-producing material.

TREATMENT: Careful feeding will overcome this condition. Warm wheat bran mashes, ground bone, beef scraps, all tend to allay the irritations of the oviduct and stimulate the secretions of albumen.

JAUNDICE

CAUSE: Obstruction of the bile duct, due to rich, nitrogenous food and insufficient exercise.

SYMPTOMS: Disease is not easily detected. The yellow color of the wattles and comb is the first symptom; the appetite is variable, the feathers appear rough and dry, the head is retracted, and the bird finally dies owing to the absorption of bile in the blood.

TREATMENT: Change food. Feed upon a vegetable diet, also give one grain of Calomel, which is particularly useful in a case of sluggish liver in poultry. Also give one grain of Pulv. Gentian Root and one grain of Bicarbonate of Soda, twice daily in feed.

MANGE

(Scabies of the Body)

CAUSE: Due to a parasite that resembles the mite.

SYMPTOMS: When the affected bird is closely examined large quantities of scales or scabs are found in the soft feathers. The appetite is poor; the bird walks slowly about showing signs of uneasiness. If the disease is allowed to run its course, the bird grows weak and eventually dies. The disease is easily transmitted from one bird to another and should be treated without delay.

TREATMENT: Disinfect roost, coops and pens with undiluted Crude Carbolic Acid. Apply to the irritations that present themselves on the body of the birds: Sulphur Ointment twice a week and feed good nourishing food as wheat bran mashes and vegetables.

PIP

(Inflammation of the Mouth)

CAUSE: Irritations, injuries, or micro-organisms. It is sometimes caused by nothing more than a dry condition of the mucous membrane due to the bird breathing through the mouth when suffering from respiratory diseases.

SYMPTOMS: Dryness of the mucous membrane of the mouth; especially the part covering the tongue, which becomes hard and ragged, forming rough edges along its sides. These dried portions become loose and partially detached from the tongue, interfering with its movements and causing more or less pain and annoyance.

TREATMENT: Do not forcibly detach these pieces, but assist nature to remove them. This can be accomplished by mixing Glycerine and Water, equal parts, and dropping into the mouth with an ordinary syringe or dropper. It is advisable to add Boracic Acid, one teaspoonful to every gallon of drinking water, which will prevent the entrance of parasites into the blood.

RED MITE

CAUSE: These grow spontaneously in favorable surroundings, as the interior of poultry houses and brooders containing numerous cracks and crevices.

SYMPTOMS: This mite is a blood-sucker; irritates the skin and sometimes causes sores to form on the body of the chick. The birds grow stupid and weak and die rapidly if not properly treated. Older fowls withstand the irritation of mites much longer, but do not thrive, or lay regularly, and will finally die if the insects become too numerous. The insect may be transmitted to horses, cattle, and even to man.

TREATMENT: Paint the roosts and spray the interior of the coops and runs with Crude Carbolic Acid, undiluted, being very careful that the solution reaches the bottoms of the cracks and crevices. Also paint the interior of brooders with the same solution.

RHEUMATISM

(Leg Weakness--Gout--Paralysis)

CAUSE: Damp coops and pens, lack of ventilation and improper food.

SYMPTOMS: Fowl refuses to stand or walk, and on examination, the legs are found to be swollen and painful, especially about the joints. In some cases suppuration of the joints takes place and they become open running sores. The bone finally becomes diseased and the fowl dies.

TREATMENT: Preventive measures are first to be considered. See that the coops and pens are clean and dry. Avoid drafts. Feed vegetables, also wheat bran mashes. Give internally Salicylic Acid, one-half grain, twice daily. When the legs are swollen and sore apply Camphorated Ointment once or twice daily.

SCALY LEG

(Scabies)

CAUSE: Due to a mite that burrows under the scales of the leg.

SYMPTOMS: White, scaly-looking scabs form about the upper part of the foot. The feet and legs become swollen and painful as the disease progresses and if not checked will result in lameness, inflammation of the joints, and the toes may slough off. Great care is necessary as the disease is very easily transmitted from one bird to another.

TREATMENT: Use boiling water or Crude Carbolic Acid, undiluted, on the perches. Wash the feet and legs with warm water and soft soap. Dry well and apply Carbolated Ointment. Repeat the above treatment every other day for a week.

SORE MOUTH

(Aphtha; Thrush)

CAUSE: A vegetable parasite called Oidium Albicans.

SYMPTOMS: Inflammation of the mucous membrane lining the mouth, throat, gullet and crop, which finally terminates in white ulcerations. Other symptoms are swelling of the head, poor appetite and a rapid loss in weight and strength.

TREATMENT: Isolate the sick from the healthy fowls. Give as much sunlight as possible, feed nourishing food, such as warm oatmeal mashes, kale, potatoes, etc. Add one grain each of Chlorate of Potash and Boracic Acid to a tablespoonful of water and give three or four times a day or oftener if they will drink it. A good disinfectant must be used to prevent the disease from spreading and I would recommend the use of undiluted Crude Carbolic Acid about the coops and poultry runs.

TUBERCULOSIS

CAUSE: This dreaded disease is caused by the Bacillus of Tuberculosis. Damp, ill-ventilated, and poorly lighted coops are favorable to the development of the disease.

SYMPTOMS: Except in advanced stages, this disease is not easily detected as it affects various organs, and considerable experience in post-mortems and a skillful use of the microscope is required to successfully diagnose a case.

TREATMENT: Preventive measures should be practiced as the disease is incurable. Do not expose the fowls to cold wet weather. See that the coops are well ventilated and lighted and feed no contaminated food.

VENT GLEET

CAUSE: Constipation is perhaps the most common cause, the hard droppings causing irritation of the vent which is followed by inflammation and suppuration of the lining membranes, rectum and oviduct.

SYMPTOMS: Frequent straining due to irritation. As the disease progresses a pus-like discharge is noticed. The disease may extend into the rectum or oviduct. The bird appears stupid, the plumage rough, the comb pale, and if not properly treated, dies a lingering death.

TREATMENT: Preventive treatment is the best. Feed green food occasionally and warm bran mashes. This prevents constipation. When the bird strains frequently and a discharge is present the following solution should be injected: Sugar of Lead, two drams; Zinc Sulphate, one dram. Mix with two quarts of water. Inject about one ounce with a syringe twice daily until the discharge has ceased.

WHITE DIARRHOEA

(Fowl Cholera)

CAUSE: Germ (Bacilli of Fowl Cholera) gaining entrance to the body through the bowels, lungs or wounds of the skin. Death results from toxic material produced while the germs are multiplying.

SYMPTOMS: All poultry, cage or wild birds are subject to this disease. The first symptoms are loss of appetite; diarrhoea is present and the discharge is almost white in color and tinged with transparent mucus. The affected bird becomes separated from the flock, seems weak and stupid and appears to be asleep; feathers are rough, the wings droop and the head is drawn in toward the body; crop is generally full, owing to improper digestion. The comb is pale and bloodless, the temperature raised from three to five degrees above normal and the bird loses weight rapidly; it may die with convulsions and cries, or without a sound or struggle.

TREATMENT: To grown fowls, give Zinc Sulphocarbolates in one-half grain doses three times a day in their food or drinking water. To chicks, dissolve thirty grains of Zinc Sulphocarbolates in two quarts of water. Saturate feed, as stale bread, etc., and give three times a day. Zinc Sulphocarbolates is an antiseptic especially prepared for septic conditions of the intestines, and very useful in treatment of White Diarrhoea and Fowl Cholera. In severe cases of diarrhoea, give Bismuth Salicylate, one grain, three times daily in feed or make into a pill with dough. When the fowls will eat, feed them clean, nitrogenous food that they can digest easily, as oatmeal mashes. It is also necessary to give them pure water to drink at all times. Disinfection of the premises is another essential factor in the treatment of this disease, and undiluted Crude Carbolic Acid is a disinfectant that we can rely upon at all times.

I cannot recommend vaccination as the serum is very difficult and expensive to produce and different breeds of birds require varying doses, therefore, vaccinating poultry for White Diarrhoea or Fowl Cholera is not attended with any great degree of success.

WORMS

CAUSE: Few fowls are entirely free from worms. The soil over which the chicks are permitted to run may be infected, or the food may contain the eggs or embryos of worms.

SYMPTOMS: The presence of worms in fowls may not be at once detected, since only a close observer would notice them in the droppings. If the birds eat well but remain poor, and the feathers appear rough and the comb and wattles pale, there is reason to suspect the existence of worms.

TREATMENT: Preventive treatment is the best. Sprinkle the runs and coops regularly with Crude Carbolic Acid, undiluted. Give two drops of Turpentine in twice this quantity of Sweet or Olive Oil. This dose should be repeated in from six to eight days so as to insure the expulsion of the newly hatched worms or those that may have survived the first treatment.

MISCELLANEOUS

Some valuable facts and figures summed up for handy reference

VALUABLE DRUGS AND THEIR DOSES FOR DOMESTIC ANIMALS

In the list of doses, oz. stands for ounce, pt. for pint, lb. for pound, gr. for grain, dr. for dram, dp. for drop.

NAME OF DRUG	CATTLE	SHEEP	HORSES	HOGS	DOGS
Alcohol	4 oz.	1-2 oz.	2-4 oz.	1-2 oz.	1-4 dr.
Alum	3-4 dr.	40 gr.	2-4 dr.	40 gr.	15 gr.
Ammonia Aromatic	2 oz.	1-2 dr.	1-2 oz.	1-2 dr.	20-60 dp.
Aniseed	1-5 oz.	1-2 dr.	1 oz.	1 dr.	15 gr.
Arnica Tincture	1 oz.	2 dr	.5-1 oz.	1 dr.	7-20 dp.
Asafetida Tincture	3 oz.	.5 oz.	2 oz.	2 dr.	1 dr.
Boracic Acid	3 dr.	20 gr.	1-3 dr.	15 gr.	8 gr.
Brandy	4 oz.	1-2 oz.	2-4 oz.	1-2 oz.	1-2 dr.
Calcium Phosphate	1 oz.	1-2 dr.	2-4 dr.	1-2 dr.	5-20 gr.
Calomel	1-2 dr.	5-20 gr.	1 dr.	5-20 gr.	1 gr.
Camphor Spirit	1 oz.	2 dr.	2-4 dr.	15 dp.	10 dp.
Carbolic Acid	1-2 dr.	10-20 dp.	.5-2 dr.	5-15 dp.	3-8 dp.
Castor Oil	1 pt.	2-4 oz.	1 pt.	2-4 oz.	1-2 dr.
Chalk	2 oz.	1-2 dr.	.5-2 oz.	1 dr.	.5-1 dr.

Charcoal 1-2 oz. 2-4 dr. 1-2 oz. 2-4 dr. 20-60 gr. Codliver Oil 3-8 oz. 3-8 dr. 2-6 oz. 2-6 dr. 1-3 dr. Copperas 2 dr. 20 gr. 1 dr. 10 gr. 4 gr. Copper Sulphate 2-4 dr. 20-30 gr. 2-4 dr. 20-30 gr. 1-2 gr. Digitalis 10-30 gr. 5-15 gr. 10-50 gr 3-10 gr. 2 gr. Epsom Salts 1 lb. 1-4 oz. .5-1 lb. 1 oz. 1-4 dr. Fowler's Solution 5 dr. 5-20 dp. 2-4 dr. 5-20 dp. 1-5 dp. Gentian 5-8 dr. 1-2 dr. 4-8 dr. 1-2 dr. 40 gr. Ginger 5-8 dr. 1-2 dr. 2-8 dr. 15-60 gr. 5-20 gr. Glauber Salts 1-1.5 lb. 1-4 dr. .5-1 lb. 1 oz. 1-4 dr. Iodide of Potash 1-2 dr. 10-25 gr. .5-2 dr. 5-20 gr. 2-8 gr. Iron Sulphate 2 dr. 25 gr. 1-2 dr. 25 gr. 4 gr. Jamaica Ginger 2 oz. .5 oz. 1 oz. .5-1 dr. 1/4-1/2 dr. Laudanum 2-5 oz. 1-4 dr. 1-4 oz. 1-2 dr. 20 dp. Lead Acetate 1 dr. 25 gr. 1 dr. 20 gr. 1-2 gr. Lime Water 4-6 oz. 2 oz. 4-6 oz. 2 oz. 1-8 dr. Linseed Oil 1-2 pt. 6-12 oz. .5-1 pt. 5-10 oz. 1 oz. Mustard 1 oz. 1-2 dr. .5-1 oz. 1-2 dr. 20 gr. Nitre 3-8 oz. 1 dr. 1-2 oz. 1 dr. 5-20 gr. Nux Vomica 2 dr. 30-40 gr. 1-2 dr. 10-20 gr. 1-2 gr. Olive Oil 1-2 pt. 3-8 dr. 1-2 pt. 2-6 dr. 2-4 oz. Pepper 2-4 dr. 15-25 gr. 1-3 dr. 10-20 gr. 4-10 gr. Peppermint Oil 30 dp. 5-8 dp. 15-30 dp. 3-7 dp. 1-5 dp. Potassium Bromide 2 oz. 2-4 dr. 1-2 oz. 2-4 dr. 5-50 gr. Quinine 1-2 dr. 5-10 gr. 50-60 gr. 5-10 gr. 1-2 gr. Rhubarb 1-2 oz. 1 dr. 1-2 oz. 1 dr. 5-10 gr. Saltpeter 1-3 dr. .5-1 dr. 2-4 dr. .5-1 dr. 2-10 gr. Soda 2 oz. 2-4 dr. 1-1.5 oz. 1-3 dr. 20-50 gr. Subnitrate of Bismuth 2 dr. 10-30 gr. 1-2 dr. 5-20 gr. 3-10 gr. Sulphur 3-4 oz. 1-2 oz. 2-4 oz. 1-2 oz. 1-4 dr. Turpentine 2 oz. 1-4 dr. 1-2 oz. 1 dr. 20-50 dp.

CHAPTER VI

RESPIRATION

The number of respirations per minute varies with the different classes of animals; as a rule, the larger the animal, the slower the respiration.

The Horse 8 to 10 Cattle 12 to 15 Sheep and Goats 12 to 20 The Dog 15 to 20 Swine 10 to 15

The rate of breathing is increased from the processes of digestion immediately after eating, or may increase from exercise.

NORMAL TEMPERATURE OF THE HORSE

From 2 to 5 years old the temperature is 100.6 degrees Fahr. From 5 to 10 years old the temperature is 100.4 degrees Fahr. From 10 to 15 years old the temperature is 100 degrees Fahr. From 15 to 20 years old the temperature is 98.4 to 100.2 degrees Fahr.

Sex appears to slightly influence temperature: Stallion 100 degrees Fahr. Mare 100.8 degrees Fahr. Gelding 100.4 degrees Fahr.

The time of day when temperature is taken is important, the lowest body temperature being at 4 a.m., and the highest at 6 p.m. New born foals' temperature will run from 102 to 104 degrees Fahr.

TEMPERATURE OF CATTLE

Normal temperature is from 101.8 to 102 degrees Fahr.

Compared with the horse, the daily variations are small.

TEMPERATURE OF SHEEP AND GOATS

In these animals the greatest variation in temperature occurs, viz.: 100.9 to 105.8 degrees Fahr. In the majority of cases the temperature probably will be between 103.6 and 104.4 degrees Fahr. The cause of this variation is unknown.

TEMPERATURE OF SWINE

The average temperature is 103.3 degrees Fahr., varying from 100.9 to 105.4 degrees Fahr.

TEMPERATURE OF THE DOG

The dog is subject to important variations depending on the external temperature; it varies from 99.5 to 101.7 degrees Fahr., although in some localities it is as high as 100.9, 101.3 and 101.7 degrees Fahr. Feeding will increase the temperature, and it is also higher toward evening.

PULSE THROBS PER MINUTE Per Minute The Horse 36 to 40 Cattle 45 to 50 Sheep and Goats 70 to 80 The Dog 70 to 80 Swine 90 to 100

The pulse in the young is much more rapid than in the adult animal; that of a foal at birth beats 100 to 102 per minute, while that of a calf will go to 130 per minute. In old age the pulsation becomes reduced and the arteries much weaker. The pulse rate in large animals is less than in smaller ones, as for instance, an elephant's pulse rate is from 25 to 28 beats per minute. The more rapid the pulse, the greater the quantity of blood in circulation.

AVERAGE PERIODS OF GESTATION OF DOMESTIC ANIMALS

Mare 11 months Ass 12 months Cow 9 months Sheep 5 months Goat 5 months Sow 3-1/2 months Bitch 9 weeks Cat 8 weeks

AVERAGE PERIOD OF INCUBATION

Chicken 20 to 22 days Geese 28 to 34 days Duck 28 to 30 days Turkey 27 to 29 days Pigeon 18 days Guinea Fowl 28 days Pheasant 25 days Ostrich 40 to 42 days Canary Bird 14 days

VETERINARY FACTS AND ADVICE TO REMEMBER

1. Cleanliness of body and surroundings is a necessity in the treatment of animals.

2. Pure air, avoiding drafts, is equally essential.

3. Light, excepting in the treatment of eye diseases, is greatly to be desired. Darkness, while soothing to the eye, tends to prolong germ life and disease.

4. Keep dry--dampness breeds disease.

5. Keep warm--in chilly weather, blanket the sick animal, hand rub limbs and bandage with woolen cloths.

6. Exercise with care--excessive and insufficient exercise are both injurious.

7. Feed with care--green grass, in medium quantity, and vegetables are cooling to the blood, easily digested and exert a slight laxative effect. Grain feed is nutritious and strengthening, but it is not required in any quantity by a

horse not working. Be sure that all feed is fresh and clean.

8. Drinking water must be pure--impure water carries many disease germs. Also avoid giving water in large quantities, especially if water is very cold.

9. Disinfection involves little time or expense, but is invaluable. Coal tar products which emulsify in water (1 part coal tar products to 50-75 parts water) should be freely and occasionally sprinkled about yards and buildings.

If only these few fundamental and common-sense principles were followed by stock raisers, a very large percentage of the ills and diseases of domestic animals would be lastingly prevented.

DRENCHING

Do not drench an animal when you can administer the necessary medicine in any other way. Drench only when absolutely necessary. A horse, in contrast with all other domestic animals, cannot breathe through its mouth. Therefore, in treating horses, drenching is especially dangerous. While drenching any animal, strangulation, pneumonia, bronchitis, etc., are liable to be caused by some of the drenching liquid escaping from the mouth into the lungs. This is a frequent occurrence in which the drenching proves to be the immediate cause of the animal's death, as in case of strangulation, or the originating cause when drenched animals later succumb to pneumonia, bronchitis, etc.

MEDICINE IN CAPSULES

In many of the treatments prescribed in the preceding pages, the use of gelatine capsules has been advised in preference to giving the medicine in any other form.

Capsules, made of gelatine, do not lie in the animal's stomach, as commonly supposed, but dissolve readily; the gelatine itself being beneficial in many cases, especially if the bowels or stomach be irritated. The animal receives the intended dose fully. It avoids any unpleasant taste. With capsule gun, or by hand, medicine in capsules is more easily and quickly given than to attempt to hold animal's head up, as is necessary when administering liquid drenches, the danger of which has been explained.

PREVENTION OF CONTAGIOUS DISEASES

Newly purchased animals or poultry should be segregated for from ten days to two weeks to give opportunity for any infectious diseases with which they may be afflicted, or have been exposed to, to fully develop. This precaution will often save the buyer from loss.

Avoid exhibiting in fairs, shows, etc., where the health of your animals might be jeopardized, especially through the presence of contagiously affected animals. If you cannot be sure proper precautions are to be taken, better forego your pride and possible prize ribbons.

HEREDITARY TENDENCIES

When breeding, it is of utmost importance to select a good female as well as male, for the least faulty conformation in either will in all probability be transferred to the offspring, viz.: an animal with a crooked hind leg is subject to bone spavin, curbs, bog spavin, thoroughpin, ring bone, etc., and is liable to transmit any of these diseases, especially if exposed to slight exertion. A tubercular cow will invariably give birth to a tubercular calf, or at any rate the calf will contract tuberculosis from the milk.

EVOLUTION OF STOCK

During the transformation which our country has undergone, and is undergoing, no one industry has experienced such marked changes as the production and raising of livestock.

At the earliest time of which we have any record, and even up to within comparatively recent years, large herds of horses and cattle ranged over our plains in a wild state. At first no attempts were made to capture or round up these herds, and later but one or two attempts per year, when the young were branded and grown animals shipped, if possible, or driven to available markets.

As the country became more thickly settled and populated these larger herds were broken up, the ranges becoming divided and fenced. With this segregation, attention to breeding and care of animals began to be practiced, gradually causing the animal's evolution from the wild to the domesticated state.

As this process of evolution progressed the animal became farther and farther removed from its natural condition of living, becoming more dependent on man for food and shelter, and with this change the animal's former vitality and power to resist disease decreased markedly.

With the advancement of agriculture, and their resultant prosperity, the farmers and settlers improved their stock by importing blooded or registered males and females, particularly the former, until today our country is second to none in the number of good conformated draft and speed horses; beef and dairy cattle; quick-maturing hogs; large wool and mutton-producing sheep, etc. Poultry has likewise been improved for both egg-laying and meat-producing qualities. The poultry industry is yet in its infancy, and offers large inducements to the practical raiser. Our importation of eggs is enormous.

The average stock raiser and poultryman has just begun to realize the value of proper care and treatment of his stock, and how much unnecessary loss can be prevented by the expenditure of a little time and even less money if given at the proper time.

Animals and poultry are subject, just as humans, to many diseases but, unfortunately, when they become ill are dependent on man to recognize the symptoms of disease and diagnose. Therefore, it behooves all owners of stock to know and practice the fundamental necessities of their animals' health, not only for the welfare of themselves, but also as an act of humanity to dumb animals.

INDEX

DISEASES OF HORSES

lameness Cold Colic, flatulent Colic, spasmodic Colic, wind Colt constipation Colt diarrhoea Conjunctivitis Constipation Constipation in colts Corns Cough Cracked heels Curb Dentistry Diarrhoea Diarrhoea in colts Dislocation of the patella Distemper Dropsy of belly Dropsy of legs Dropsy of sheath Dropsy of udder Eczema Emphysema of the lungs Epizootic catarrh Eye diseases Failure to breed Farcy Filariae Fistula of foot Fistulous withers Flatulent colic Forage poisoning Founder Galls Gastrophilis Glanders Grease heels Haemopis Heaves Hernia, inguinal Horse dentistry Inflammation of the brain Inflammation of the membrane of nictitans Influenza Inguinal hernia Lampas Laryngitis Leeches Lock jaw Lung fever Lymphangitis Mange Monday Morning disease Mud fever Nasal catarrh Nasal gleet Navel rupture Navel string infection Navicular disease Nettle rash Open joint Oxyuris curvilis Palesade worm Petchial fever Pharyngitis Pink eye Pin worm Pleurisy Pneumonia Poll evil Purpura haemorrhagica Quittor Red worm Rheumatism Ring bone Round worm Rupture, scrotal Scabies Scrotal rupture Septicaemia Shoe boil Side bones Sore throat Spasmodic colic Spavin, bog Spavin, bone Splints Staggers Stifle joint lameness String halt Strongulus armatus Strongulus tetracanthus Supernumerary teeth Surfeit Sweeny Tapeworm Teeth, supernumerary Teeth, wolf Tenia Tetanus Thoroughpin Thread-like worm Thrush Umbilical hernia Umbilical pyemia Urtecaria Wind colic Wind galls Wolf teeth Worm, maw Worm, palesade Worm, pin Worm, red Worm, round Worm, tape Worm, thread Worm, thread-like Wounds

DISEASES OF CATTLE

Abdominal hernia Abdominal rupture Abnormal Calving Abortion, contagious Abortion, non-contagious Abscesses Absence of milk Actinomycosis Acute cough Afterbirth retention Amaurosis of the eye Anthrax Apoplexy, parturient Ascities Bacterial dysentery Bag Inflammation Barrenness Big head Black leg Black quarter Bleeding Bloating Blood poison Blood suckers Bloody flux Bloody flux in calves Bloody milk Blue milk Brain congestion Bronchitis Bronchitis verminous Calf cholera Calf scours Calving Casting the withers Cataract of the eye Catarrh Chapped teats Choking Chronic cough Chronic dysentery Colic Congestion of the brain Congestion of the lungs Congestion of the spinal cord Congestion of the udder Conjunctivitis Contagious abortion Cough Cow pox Cud chewing Dehorning Diarrhoea Dropsy Dysentery Eczema Epizootica eczema Ergot poisoning Ergotism Eversion of the womb Eye inflammation Eyelid laceration Failure to breed

Fluke, liver Fluke, lung Foot and mouth disease Foot rot Foul in foot Founder Garget Grub Hard milkers Hematuria Hemorrhage Hernia, abdominal Hollow horn Indigestion Infectious abortion Infectious aphtha Inflammation of the bag Inflammation of the eye Inflammation of the heart sack Inflammation of the kidneys Inflammation of the penis Inflammation of the womb Joint ill Jones disease Kidney inflammation Laceration of the eyelid Laminitis Laryngitis Leeches Leucorrhea Liver fluke Loss of cud Lumpy jaw Lung congestion Lung fever Lung fluke Mammitis, simple Mange Measly beef Milk fever Navel ill Non-contagious abortion Obstruction of the esophagus Paralysis Parturient apoplexy Penis Inflammation Pericarditis Pharyngitis Physiology of rumination Pneumonia Pyemia Red Water Retained afterbirth Rheumatism Ring worm Round worm Rupture, abdominal Scabies Scum over the eye Septicaemia Sore throat Spinal cord congestion Stringy milk Suppression of milk Tape worm Teats chapped Texas fever Ticks Tuberculosis Twisted stomach worm Udder congestion Umbilical Pyemia Umbilical Septicemia Variola Verminous bronchitis Warts Warbles Whites White scours in calves Wolf in the tail Womb inflammation Wooden tongue Worm, lung Worm, round Worm, stomach Worm, tape

DISEASES OF SWINE

Abortion Administration of medicine Bag inflammation Black tooth Blood poisoning Bronchitis Castration Catarrh Choking Cholera, hog Cold in the head Congestion, kidney Diarrhoea in young pigs Heat stroke Hind quarter paralysis Hog, administration of medicine Hog cholera Hog lice Hog regulator and tonic Indigestion Inflammation, bag Inflammation, lung Inguinal rupture Jaundice Kidney congestion Kidney worms Lice on hogs Lung fever Lung inflammation Lung worm Mange Nasal catarrh Navel rupture Nettle rash Paralysis of the hind quarters Pig diarrhoea Pig scours Piles Pin worm Pleurisy Prolapse of the anus Pyemia Regulator and tonic Rheumatism Rickets Round worm Rupture, inguinal Rupture, navel Rupture, scrotal Rupture, umbilical Septicemia Scours in pigs Scrotal rupture Sore feet Sore mouth Sows eating their young Sun stroke Thorn headed worm Thumps Tonic and regulator Urticaria Worm, kidney Worm, lung Worm, pin Worm, round Worm, thorn headed Worm, whip Yellows

DISEASES OF SHEEP AND GOATS

Abortion Acute indigestion Acute typanitis Apoplexy, pulmonary Black scours Bloating Bronchitis Catarrh Cold in the head Congestion of the liver Congestion of the lung Congestion of the udder Diarrhoea Dysentery Dyspepsia Foot rot Forage poisoning Foul in foot Garget Gastritis, verminous Gid Grub in the head Head grubs Head maggot Hoven Indigestion Indigestion, acute Inflammation of the liver Inflammation of the udder Jaundice Lamb disease Liver congestion Liver fluke Liver inflammation Louse fly Lung congestion Lung fever Lung worm Mange Pneumonia Poisoning, forage Pulmonary apoplexy Scab Scours, black Strongylosis Sturdy Tick Typanitis, acute Udder, congestion of Udder, inflammation of Verminous bronchitis Verminous gastritis Worm, lung

DISEASES OF POULTRY

Abortion Abscesses of the feet. Air sac mite Apoplexy of the brain Aptha Ascites Baldness Beak and throat obstruction Black head Body lice Body scabies Brain apoplexy Bronchitis Bronchitis verminous Bruises of the feet. Bumblefoot Catarrh Catarrh of the crop Chicken pox Cholera of the fowl Congestion of the liver Constipation Corns Crop impaction Diarrhoea Diarrhoea, white Difficult laying Diphtheria Diphtheritic roup Double yolked eggs Dropsy Egg bound Egg eating Egg incomplete Eggs with two yolks Eggs without shells Enteritis Favus Feather eating Feather pulling Feeding of young poultry Fowl cholera Gapes Gastro intestinal catarrh Gout Head lice Hemorrhage of the brain How to feed young poultry Impaction of the crop Incomplete egg Infectious entero hepatitis of turkeys Inflammation of the crop Inflammation of the mouth Intestinal obstruction Jaundice Leg weakness Lice, body Lice, head Liver congestion Mange Mite, red Mouth inflammation Obstruction of the beak and throat Obstruction of the bile duct Obstruction of the crop Obstruction of the intestines Obstruction of the oviduct Paralysis of the crop Paralysis of the legs Pip Pulmonary congestion Red mite Rheumatism Roup, diphtheritic Scabies of the body Scabies of the legs Scaly leg Soft shelled eggs Sore head Sore mouth Throat and beak obstruction Thrush Tuberculosis Vent gleet Verminous tracheo bronchitis Warts White diarrhoea Worms

MISCELLANEOUS

Average Period of Gestation Average Period of Incubation Deposit or Investment Table Drenching of Animals Evolution of Stock Hereditary Tendencies Medicine in Capsules Normal Purse Throbs Normal Respiration Normal Temperature Prevention of Contagious Diseases Six Per Cent Interest Table Table of Valuable Drugs and their Doses Veterinary Facts and Advice to Remember

###

www.ingramcontent.com/pod-product-compliance
Lightning Source LLC
Chambersburg PA
CBHW070855180526
45168CB00005B/1828